The God of the Low Places

Finding God in Depression

by

Karen Maximin

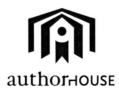

authorHOUSE

1663 LIBERTY DRIVE, SUITE 200
BLOOMINGTON, INDIANA 47403
(800) 839-8640
www.authorhouse.com

First published by AuthorHouse 09/11/04

ISBN: 1-4184-6724-3 (e)
ISBN: 1-4184-6723-5 (sc)

Library of Congress Control Number: 2004093771

Printed in the United States of America
Bloomington, Indiana

This book is printed on acid-free paper.

With love and gratitude to my production team:
Susan J. Early, editorial director
Michael R. Moscynski, artistic director
Thomas J. Moscynski, marketing director

Table of Contents

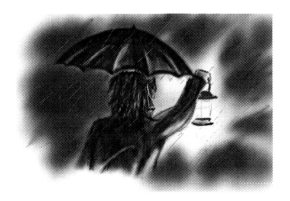

1. What am I seeking?

In the Bible, we often encounter God on physical heights. He gave the law to Moses on the top of a mountain. Jerusalem, his holy city, was likewise on top of a mountain. Even the crucifixion of his Son, the lowest point in the relationship between God and us, took place on the Hill of Golgotha, also known as Calvary.

Emotionally and spiritually, we tend to worship God from the "high places" as well. When we are feeling good, the sun shining and the clouds puffy, we sing out "Glory be..." with rejoicing. Peace, love, joy—and all the gifts of the Spirit—are ours, and we love Father, Son, and Holy Spirit, and neighbor as well.

On the other hand, depression is a low place emotionally. Not only are we unable to find our own feelings of love, we are sometimes unable to feel that God cares at all. This book is about finding God in depression. He is our hope for the future. He is still there when our feelings of joy are gone. More importantly, he still loves. He always loves. Guaranteed.

I can't give driving directions like Mapquest for finding God. I include a few landmarks from my journey which began with my first diagnosis twenty years ago and from the journeys of those I have known along the way.

Before I make the journey of seeking God in depression, I have to know what it is I am looking for. People speak of trying to find God in ordinary circumstances. My circumstances are not ordinary. I have an illness called depression. I have a special need of God.

Something hurts, but I don't know what that something is. It's not like a toothache that I can point to. I am immobilized. I have some of the clinical symptoms of depression which include (lists vary):

- sadness
- weight loss or gain
- physical symptoms that do not respond to treatment
- irritability
- fatigue
- change in sleep patterns
- loss of interest or pleasure in activities
- loss of concentration, memory
- suicidal thoughts.

What I want is to be able to get through the day—to get past the struggle to move, the lost time when my mind goes away, the sudden anxiety attack when I am doing something harmless like reading the funnies. I am so glad when the day is almost over, but then I have to get through the night—the restlessness, the wandering through a darkened house or apartment, the racing thoughts, until finally the night is over and I face another day to get through.

Can God take me out of this down spiral? Will he?

I want to know God's role in my life. Is this suffering a random chance occurrence, or is it part of God's plan? Is there a higher purpose so that he will at some point bring good from this?

I want to find God so I can ask him if he's angry. Is this a punishment for my sins? I don't remember having been that bad. Even if I was, what happened to forgiveness? For that matter, when I am depressed, it feels as though I am not following God's plan. Is my depression a sin?

I want the God of peace to guide me, to comfort me. I feel like I am no longer even on planet Earth. I have been removed unwillingly to a new planet where nothing looks the same, not the sky, not the ground, not the plants. I am alone on this planet. Even the gravity is different. Sometimes it weighs me down, but at other times each step causes me to bounce higher. Is God with me on this strange planet? I want him to find me and help me.

Beyond all this, I want to find God for the sake of God. My heart was made by him to love him. Jesus died for my sins and calls me brother or sister [Hebrews 2:11-12]. He sent his Spirit. I've been taught these things, but I want to feel them. I don't know if that's possible in depression, but I feel a need to know God more intimately.

Am I seeking healing? And what do I mean by healing? I pray for healing, even though I am not sure what it will look like. For example, suppose I accidentally cut my finger. It bleeds a little until I wash it and bandage it. Using it or putting pressure on it hurts. Each day the finger hurts less while the wound closes up. In very short time it is healed. It looks the same except maybe for a thin white scar. It functions the same. It is, as they say, good as new.

Healing from depression is different. Depending on how much time has elapsed. and the severity of the depression, we may not be able to go back to the way we were before. When I have fallen off the edge of a cliff, I don't expect to be able to scale its sheer face to get back to where I was. Healing begins when I step forward—even though bruised and hurting—to find a new path, even a new destination. Depression is a bruising, punishing, humiliating experience, but it is only terminal if we let it be.

In the miracles recorded in Scripture, Jesus restored completely:

> When they arrived at Bethsaida, they brought to him a blind man and begged him to touch him. He took the blind man by the hand and led him outside the village. Putting spittle on his eyes he laid his hands on him and asked, "Do you see anything?" Looking up he replied, "I see people looking like trees and walking!" Then he laid hands on his eyes a second time and he saw clearly; his sight was restored and he could see everything distinctly.
>
> Mark 8:22-25

Jesus used his spittle to heal—how odd! And we thought the meds were invasive. The man was not healed all at once. This is a lesson to us that healing can come in stages. We must not despair if we are in the tree-walking stage. In a later chapter we explore more extensively what it means to be healed.

Am I seeking support from others? Family and friends usually mean well, but they can be confused, pessimistic, discouraged, and discouraging. They may feel a need to take control of our lives, to make our decisions for us, to rearrange our kitchens for us just at the time when we are least able to cope with rearrangements. To be fair, there have been times when I have needed someone to take charge and see that I got help, times when I felt as if I were lying with a broken leg in the middle of the street and could not get help for myself.

At any rate, they don't know any better. Somebody always has an Aunt Nellie who lived in an earlier generation, who was taken away by the men in white coats and never came back. (It happened to my grandmother.) Now the length of stay in a hospital is often less than a week. There isn't time to make a string art picture in OT. Such a pity. And there are fewer hospitalizations. Some point to the improved medications as reason. Certainly managed care has its influence. We are primarily out in the community, and the community doesn't know how to relate to us.

On the other extreme are the people who don't recognize that I have changed. They say, "You look okay to me." It tends to make me want to hang my head a little lower to prove them wrong. I am afraid they will expect of me more than I can give. Of course I look okay. Did you expect I would have snakes for hair like Medusa?

Fortunately some people are between these two extremes. They may not understand what is happening, but they are willing to try to stay with us.

Addiction.

Half the people with a mental illness are addicted to alcohol or to drugs such as cocaine. The illness and the addiction together are a double whammy.

Both need healing. The idea that by treating one, the other will go away has been proved to be false. If I had a broken arm and a broken leg, I wouldn't expect that putting a cast on the leg would heal the arm as well. The problems interfere with each other. The broken arm keeps me from using crutches to get around on the broken leg.

In addiction, the brain is becoming addicted to itself. The substance (or activity, such as gambling) causes the brain's pleasure center (the limbic system) to produce dopamine. It sends a pleasure message. The brain realigns itself to send a message to seek more. This is why a person can be completely detoxified and still have cravings days or even months later. The message is not coming from the body. It is coming from the brain.

Successful treatment programs such as Alcoholics Anonymous and Narcotics Anonymous reprogram the brain. They include reliance on God (a higher power), accountability to others (the meetings), and a new message (the Twelve Steps) to replace the old. Unfortunately some AA programs discourage the use of psychotropic medications, making these programs unsuitable for persons with mental illness.

Some Dual Recovery programs exist. For more information on Dual Recovery programs, see http// draonline.org or call 877-883-2332 toll-free.

Motivation to build a new life.

What am I seeking? Why am I seeking anything at all? We have to have a reason. We can't push a limp string. It rolls up into a little ball. We must be pulled forward by some motivation, some reason for trying.

The most powerful reason is that it can happen. We can feel better. We can be interested in life again. Many have done it. For example, I have been to consumer conferences. Virtually every state has them, often with scholarship money available. I have found consumers at all stages of getting on with their lives.

More consumer experiences can be found online, for example at mhrecovery.com. Above all, we have to believe it can happen. We get that from each other. Many times I have talked to people whose goal was to stay out of the hospital. The real question is: And do what? Out of the wide range of possible motivations, some include:

- to make enough money to buy a car;
- to have family life restored;
- to finish school;
- to travel without fear;
- to write a book.

If we set our faces toward our goals (to use a Biblical expression), there is no guarantee that we will wind up there, but we will move in a positive direction. Do I believe that God has a path for each of us? Yes, I firmly believe he created us with purpose, and will lead us by a pillar of cloud just as he led the Israelites out of Egypt. It will not happen by sitting at the end of the path and praying, expecting it will carry us forward like a moving sidewalk at the airport. We embark on the path not knowing for sure where it will take us. There will be blind alleys where we must retrace our steps, but I believe that the Lord will lead us to our ultimate goal. I have come so far already.

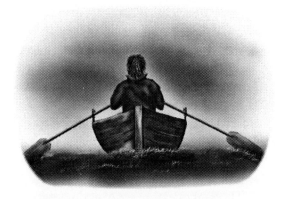

2. Faith, hope, and love.

God's gifts are like flowers from a secret admirer. We know there is someone who cares, who gives freely. Although we don't always recognize that God is the source, he gives us gifts of faith, hope and love because he cares for us.

Faith.

What does faith look like? How do I know I have faith? I believe in God, but I doubt myself. I know that God exists, one God in three Persons, but could I be described as a person of faith? I look in the mirror to see if I "have" faith. I don't see a halo. I'm wearing a crucifix, but anyone can buy a crucifix and put it on. Faith is internal. It is a gift. I need to relax and let it happen.

Faith comes from experience. For instance, I buy a particular brand of cake mix. My mother-in-law first recommended it to me. (God rest her soul.) As I tried different types—the yellow and the German chocolate and the frostings—I found that even I could get good results from that brand. I grew more confident. Similarly with faith. We hear about it from others and try it for ourselves. As I turned to God for different reasons, and as he responded, I grew more confident in the relationship.

Jesus likened faith to a mustard seed:

> "Amen, I say to you, if you have faith the size of a mustard seed, you will say to this mountain, 'Move from here to there,' and it will move. Nothing will be impossible for you."
>
> Matthew 17:20

A mustard seed is tiny, smaller than the size of an "o" on this page, yet that speck of life uses air, water, nutrients in the soil, and sunlight to grow to be a large shrub, taller than a person. Where does it come from? If I were to take air, water, and soil without the seed, the best I could make would be a mud pie. The mustard plant has a definite shape with distinct leaves and blooms, not a juniper or a rhododendron but a mustard plant. It is a miracle. Similarly our faith does not just grow but is in itself a miracle of grace with form of its own.

Faith moves mountains. To be depressed is to be in a low place, surrounded by mountains of despair and discouragement with ourselves, misunderstanding and stigma from others. Our faith tells us that we can move these mountains piece by piece.

Faith goes beyond believing in an eternal God somewhere in the sky. Faith incorporates a trust in the fidelity and love of that God. It means knowing that this God wants us to be with him for all eternity, that he will always provide choices which make that possible, and that he will give us the grace to make those choices if we accept it. To have faith means to believe that God wants us. Me. Us. Each of us. God is love.

Faith is like an antibiotic, a natural aid to healing from depression. People can recover from pneumonia without antibiotics, but usually it takes longer, and not all make it. Similarly people without a faith life recover from mental illness, but the odds are in favor of those with an active faith:

> . .. a growing body of literature has begun to suggest that religion may also be associated with more rapid clinical improvement or enhanced mental health care outcomes.[1]

At the desolate times, having faith is like being in a rowboat in the middle of the ocean. I am buoyed up. It's better than treading water. In a storm I could still drown in human terms, but in God's terms I am safe. He will not let go.

> Can a mother forget her infant,
> be without tenderness for the child of her womb?
> Even should she forget,
> I will never forget you.

> Isaiah 49: 15

Clergy are not always prepared to deal with the problems of depression. I remember telling one priest that God felt distant. His belittling response was, "If God is distant, who moved?" St. Teresa of Avila wrote more empathetically of depression:

> At such a time, faith, like all the other virtues, is quite numbed and asleep. It is not lost, for the soul has a firm belief in what is held by the Church; but though it can testify with the mouth, it seems in other respects to be oppressed and stupefied, and it feels as if it knows God only as something of which it has heard from afar off. So lukewarm does its love become that, if it hears Him spoken of, it listens, believing that He is Who He is, because this is held by the Church, but it retains no memory of its own experiences of Him...[2]

At these times it is sufficient merely to "practice" faith—to read scripture, go to church, address our prayers to the wind. God has not gone away, nor has he forgotten us. We are in a rowboat in the middle of the ocean.

Hope.

We hope for good. "Expect" means something is likely to happen, good or bad. Some days the market analysts expect the Dow-Jones to go up, and some days they expect it to go down. A "wish" is fanciful, something we don't realistically expect, like wishing to win the lottery. Hope is both concrete and transcendent. Like wishing, we hope for something good. Like expecting, what we hope for is possible.

Faith augments hope. With faith we believe in God's promise of goodness, a purposeful act from a supreme being. Without faith, we are hoping for a random act of chance, a toss of the dice.

We don't always know what we are hoping for. We hope to leave depression behind, but we can't necessarily envision what will be ahead. As St. Paul wrote,

> For in hope we were saved. Now hope that sees for itself is not hope. For who hopes for what one sees? But if we hope for what we do not see, we wait with endurance.

Romans 8:24-25

Well-meaning people can have the effect of robbing us of our hope, like taking a scrub brush and erasing our rainbows from the sky. I can remember during one hospitalization that a doctor told me I would be depressed for the rest of my life. I told him I'd prove him wrong in a year. That was almost twenty years ago. I don't remember his name, and I have no idea where he is now. I still take meds, and there are occasional mild symptoms to deal with, but I don't consider myself sick in the sense that he meant.

We can hope for big things or small. I hope the sun will come out. Sooner or later it will, and it will lift my spirits. I have hoped to get a job, to come off disability. I stood before an outdoor statue of St. Joseph and prayed to be able to return to work. It took a few more years, but it happened. Patience is a slow form of hope.

Love.

We use the word "love" to mean fellowship, commitment, romantic love, dependency/codependency, sexual attraction, spiritual bond, and a craving for pizza. Whole books have been written trying to define love.

At the same time, we each have a soul which already knows what love is, wordlessly, without Webster's. It learned it from the steadfast love of the Father, from Jesus who was the Word among us, and from the infusion of the Spirit. If we only make the choice, the commitment to say "I love," our soul knows what we mean and how to respond. If I make the choice to say, "I love God," or "I love the kids," my soul understands and loves.

It is possible to love a cat or a symphony or a memory in some senses of the word. Maybe it is our starting place. We as people of depression must thaw our hearts any way we can, but the ultimate goal is to enter into trusting relationships.

Try to love. That was the advice a priest gave me about healing, probably the best advice anybody gave me. It startled me a little. Did I love? I had to admit that my love had its element of complacency if not outright hibernation. As I entered depression, I became increasingly focused on my own needs, as one in a burning building focuses on an exit. And I have to admit that—for whatever reason—love does not come spontaneously to me (with a few exceptions). I am indeed a person who has to try to love, and I find that effort to be a key to the exit from depression.

St. Paul didn't so much define love as to say what love looks like in the following oft-quoted passage. I will insert it phrase by phrase to allow each thought to be reflected upon:

> Love is patient;
> love is kind.
> It is not jealous,
> [love] is not pompous,
> it is not inflated,

it is not rude,
it does not seek its own interests,
it is not quick-tempered,
it does not brood over injury,
it does not rejoice over wrongdoing but rejoices with
the truth.
It bears all things, believes all things, hopes all things,
endures all things.

1 Corinthians 13:4-7

I have to admit I am still trying to love. I can be impatient (especially with myself), jealous, self-seeking, to name a few. One help in the effort is a prayer a woman taught me:

Lord, today please hold my hand.
Help me to love and to understand.

It is a child's prayer, but then we are all children. She was probably in her sixties and had said the prayer her whole life. She had an inner glow. I have been saying it ever since I met her. I don't glow, but I feel oriented toward trying to love.

An example of boundless love is the story of the Prodigal Son (Luke 15:11-32). The younger son asked for his share of the father's wealth. This son then squandered it all on loose living. Finding himself broke and hungry, he returned to his father's home with the intention of asking his father to take him on as a hired hand. His father saw him approaching from afar and called for robe, ring, and sandals—all signifying exalted position—and called for the fatted calf to be prepared for a feast. So great was his love for his son that he did not brood over what his son had done, only rejoiced that his son was back.

There is a second story within this story, that of the older son who stayed home and helped his father. His protest was that it wasn't fair. He'd been the obedient one, the helpful one, and he'd never had so much as a kid goat. His father tried to explain that this son was loved as well, but the older son remained jealous. He wouldn't go in to the party. It just didn't seem fair.

Love isn't fair. Another parable dealing with fairness is in Matthew 20:1-16. Jesus told of a wealthy landowner who hired people to work in his fields. Men who didn't have jobs would wait in a certain part of the city for people to hire them. The landowner hired some workers in the morning and agreed to pay them the usual daily wage. He hired more workers at noon, at midafternoon, and later in the day.

When the day was done, the landowner paid the last group first and gave them a full day's wages, even though they had only worked about an hour. When he came to pay the group who had worked in the fields all day, they expected more. He gave them also a day's wages. When they complained, he pointed out that this was the amount they had agreed upon. It was his money, and he could be generous if he pleased.

In our society of time clocks and carefully negotiated labor contracts, this parable goes against everything we think of as being right. No matter how we try to justify it, the fact remains that the first group did more work for the same pay. The owner of the vineyard made a point of paying the last first, of letting the first group of workers see that the last were paid a full day's wages. They had every reason to expect that they would be paid more since they had worked harder.

Presumably this parable is about those who were called later to the Church, specifically Gentiles, and received the same reward of eternal life from a generous Father. But we will take the liberty of looking at it from a different level. As the older brother of the Prodigal Son observed, love isn't fair. The parable of the vineyard is saying to learn to accept what doesn't seem fair. Love isn't fair. As with the parable, we can look at a relationship six different ways and not be able to justify it as fair and square. Only when we realize the infinite dimensions of love can we let go of the yardstick.

God loves, but the way God distributes his gifts isn't fair. Some people can swing a bat and make millions. Me, I get depression. But my depression has helped me to love God, to see him in my life. Listening to post-game interviews, I learn that many ballplayers have known God through their gifts.

Love is beyond being fair. It is patient, kind. There is no limit to love's forbearance, to its trust, its hope, its power to endure. Love is the fuel that keeps us going, the meaning in our lives.

> Help me to love the leper
>> the ugly, the deformed, the twisted;
>> the loud, the obnoxious, the rude;
>> the unwashed, the unkempt, the slovenly;
>> the gloomy, the morose, the sullen;
>> the self-righteous, the sanctimonious, the
>> arrogant;
>> the hateful, the petty, the cruel.

Help me to love those who unsettle me,
  those who intimidate me,
  those who thwart me,
  those who irritate me,
  those who inundate me.
Help me to see that they are in God's image
  even though they appear unlovable,
  especially because they appear unlovable,
  they need to be loved
  and I need to love.
  Help me to love the leper,
  through Christ from whom is all love.

private prayer

Not only have I known most of these, I have been most of these at one time or another. To know is to love. We have faith when we know and love God. We have hope because he loves us. In the end, it is all about love.

Truth.

Some things I regard as absolute truth, for example, God in the persons of Father, Son, and Spirit. On our human plane, the truth gets a little muddier. We all confront questions of truth every day. An advertiser promises us the best car for the best deal. Our politicians tell us that "tactical air strikes" don't hurt anybody. Come again?

When I try to polarize my decisions, I find myself grappling for an absolute truth that doesn't exist. For example, often I have wondered whether it was better to push forward or pull back. Do I push ahead trying to get things done, making commitments to force myself into action? It seems that I had done too much of that, and getting stressed out was part of what made me sick. Then do I pull back, sink into inactivity, try to give my mind space to heal? My fear is that I would become trapped in ennui, that my mind would become flabby like an unused muscle, and that I would never function again. .

As I said, it is a question I asked myself often. In the meantime I muddled along with a little pushing forward here, a little pulling back there. I finally realized that the truth was somewhere in between, not on one side of the pendulum or the other.

In mental illness, truth is an elusive quality. To use a phrase, occasionally it's all in our minds. Hallucinations involve sensory distortions, seeing things that are not real, hearing voices, smelling things not there. Delusions, on the other hand, are confusions of thought such as thinking one is being followed or targeted. Both are more common in other mental illnesses, such as schizophrenia, but they can occur in depression. To a limited extent, I've been there. More common are the smaller self-myths, for example, feelings of worthlessness.

We don't always know what to believe about ourselves. My first psychiatrist (whom I called the dragonlady) told me I was depressed on the first visit. I suppose she felt she had to meet any denial head on. And I did deny it. To my mind, being depressed meant being in a bad mood, feeling low, deliberately being difficult. As far as I was concerned, I wasn't having any feelings at all (more denial). I had come to her because I had stopped being able to get things done, and it was stressing me out.

We all know of course how much stigma and misunderstanding there is around mental illness. Part of the reason for my vehement denial was that I didn't know the clinical meaning of the term she used. To me it implied wimpy, if not despicable. Because of stigma—and my own misunderstanding—to accept the term meant to label myself an undesirable. I was like the character described by Sartre:

> Something has happened to me, I can't doubt it any more. It came as an illness does, not like an ordinary certainty, not like anything evident. It came cunningly, little by little. . . .
>
> For instance, there is something new about my hands, a certain way of picking up my pipe or fork. Or else it's the fork which now has a certain way of having itself picked up, I don't know....
>
> There are a great number of suspicious noises in the streets, too.
>
> So a change has taken place during these last few weeks. But where? It is an abstract change without object. Am I the one who has changed? If not, then it is this room, this city and this nature; I must choose.

Nausea, Jean-Paul Sartre, p. 4

Sartre framed the dilemma well. It seems as though the world has changed, but only my own world, not the world around me. The only other possibility is that I have changed in the way I perceive the world, but that would mean that I am not in touch with reality, which is not acceptable. It would mean there was something wrong with me. Some people choose not to think of themselves as mentally ill.

It's okay to be crazy. I use the world's term here because it is the world's term we have to reconcile with.

We have to learn to distinguish what is real only to us, what thoughts are safe to act on. For this insight it is good to have discerning persons, for example, a clergy who believes in mind-experiences or a therapist who believes in spiritual experiences, as well as friends who can be relied on for both truth and understanding.

St. Paul described the various roles played by different people in the church:

> To each individual the manifestation of the Spirit is given for some benefit. To one is given through the Spirit the expression of wisdom; to another the expression of knowledge according to the same Spirit; to another faith by the same Spirit; to another gifts of healing by the one Spirit; to another mighty deeds; to another prophecy; to another discernment of spirits; to another varieties of tongues; to another interpretation of tongues. But one and the same Spirit produces all of these, distributing them individually to each person as he wishes.
>
> 1 Corinthians 12:7-11

To one person is given the visions, to another the gift of being able to discern whether those visions are valid. By visions we mean both the creative ideas and the impulses to create or destroy. Ernest Hemingway and Virginia Woolf were both bipolar, both persons of creative genius. Yet they also had in common that they killed themselves. End of gifts. We cannot be our own discerning persons.

What is truth? We pray to know God's answer, and connect with people whom we can trust to give us truth.

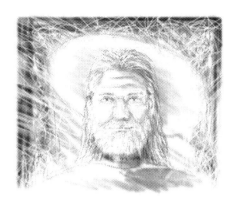

3. Who is God?

God is a very old man with a long beard who sits on a throne above the clouds. He can be cranky and lob thunderbolts, but he might also send a beatific beam of light through the clouds to bless some soul.

Or God is an abstract pulse of energy vibrating through the universe at a molecular level, maybe like the Force in Star Wars.

Or God is a clockwinder who created the universe like a precise piece of machinery. He set it in motion and went away to let it run itself.

Or God is.

I tend to personalize God although I know he is more. I randomly address any of the three Persons of the Trinity—Father, Son, and Spirit. I might relate more to one than another at any given time.

For comparison's sake, consider a chimpanzee's concept of humankind. Chimps are pretty smart, can be taught lots of things, even a couple of hundred words in sign language. Yet a chimp has absolutely no comprehension of how the human mind works because the human mind is so much further advanced. Picture trying to explain a tea bag to a chimp, how the tea was grown, how it wound up first in the little bag and then in the box, how in the store it was exchanged for dollar bills and coins.

We are like that. We don't know how God does what he does. As far as we are from the chimp's understanding, so far is comprehension of God beyond us and then some. It's the difference between finite and infinite.

We all have images and concepts of God, some rudimentary from Sunday School, some more sophisticated and intuitive. We have been taught attributes of God— goodness, love, omniscience, omnipotence. He is too big to put a dictionary definition on. He just is.

> "But," said Moses to God, "when I go to the Israelites and say to them, 'The God of your fathers has sent me to you,' if they ask me, 'What is his name?' what am I to tell them?" God replied, "I am who am." Then he added, "This is what you shall tell the Israelites: I AM sent me to you."
>
> Exodus 3:13-14

Even though we know God is Spirit, we have been describing God in human shape for a very long time:

face: The LORD let his face shine upon you, and be gracious to you!

Numbers 6:25

ear: incline your ear to me, make haste to rescue me!

Psalm 31:3a

Such imagery helps our minds to know God. All too often when I pray I have an image of a steel wall—gray, smooth, impenetrable. I try to remind myself that God is smiling. He is not impassive. He is delighted to hear from me. He sent his Son to show me his face.

Try to be loved. Not lovable—not cute and cuddly— but loved as I am, for who I am, for that is how God loves me. It is not enough to try to love. I have to believe God's love is there, individual and unfailing.

See what love the Father has bestowed on us that we may be called the children of God.

1 John 3:1

I can remember an evening shortly before my third hospitalization. I knew I had stopped functioning again. That in itself was depressing. I lay face down on my bed and despaired. When would I ever get out of it, get away from the sickness? As I lay there, I felt the hand of God touch my right shoulder, not a physical touch, and yet I was so sure he was there. "Courage, daughter."

God is like the oxygen in the atmosphere. It is in every cell of our bodies, giving us life, and yet it is in the air

23

all around us. God is his son Jesus who walked with us and died for us. Jesus also used metaphors to describe himself. In the Gospel of John he said "I am" seven times:

> "I am the bread of life; whoever comes to me will never hunger, and whoever believes in me will never thirst."

> John 6:35

> "I am the light of the world. Whoever follows me will not walk in darkness, but will have the light of life."

> John 8:12

> "I am the gate. Whoever enters through me will be saved, and will come in and go out and find pasture."

> John 10:9

> "I am the good shepherd, and I know mine and mine know me."

> John 10:14

> "I am the resurrection and the life; whoever believes in me, even if he dies, will live, and everyone who lives and believes in me will never die."

> John 11:25-26

> "I am the way and the truth and the life. No one comes to the Father except through me."

> John 14:6

"I am the vine, you are the branches. Whoever remains in me and I in him will bear much fruit, because without me you can do nothing."

John 15:5

With each metaphor, there is a promise. With each there is love, because God is love. It is not so important to define God as to define a relationship with him. Who is God? The One who loves me unconditionally.

Clergy are often the initial point of contact for a person seeking help for mental illness. They are discreet, bound by confidentiality. They are good listeners, approachable, often someone already familiar to the person seeking help. The person may feel overwhelmed and have a need to turn to God.

I was seeking a confessor. I wasn't getting anything done, a big sin in my book, felt incapable of getting anything done, concentration shot. I wasn't sleeping. I was tired. When Holy Week came, I planned to go to a penance service across town where nobody knew me. I was that ashamed. I figured if I could confess my sins of idleness, have a priest tell me to get my act together, I would snap out of it. Unfortunately, that Tuesday evening it started to snow. By 7:30 the flakes were coming thick and furious, and traveling across town was out of the question.

I despaired. I prayed silently. In that silence I felt God telling me to talk to Fr. Joe, the associate pastor of my own church. The next morning there were two feet of snow in the driveway, an April anomaly. I tackled it. The neighbor kid tried to help. Finally I called for a truck with a blade. I was determined to get out. I had made an appointment for three with Fr. Joe.

When I got to the church, the lot had been scraped. Fr. Joe's red car was alone. I pulled up next to it. From the doorway

*I heard piano music and followed it. Fr. Joe was playing ragtime
on a piano in one of the classrooms. We went to his office, a long
narrow room with two chairs at the end toward the window. Fr.
Joe's collar was open.*

*I started with the ritual words, "Bless me Father, for I
have sinned." He waited. I jumped in, told him I wasn't getting
anything done, was wasting God's time. He declined to be an
authority figure.*

*As the April-strong sun poured in through the windows,
broken only by a few hanging plants in lackluster health, we
talked about God. We talked about my life and where God fit in,
as clockwinder or as a more personal God.*

"Lady, you're about to break," Fr. Joe said.

*His words cut through me like a knife, but I denied them.
"No, I'm tough. Tough and stubborn and independent. And I
like running my own life. I don't want God to run it." We talked
some more about refocusing, extricating from over-involvement,
and he gave me a St. Francis prayer card to meditate on for
penance. He also gave me absolution and a hug.*

*Nevertheless I left angry. God was asking too much. I
stopped in the grocery for milk and ran into the woman who had
co-chaired the fall Book Fair with me at the school. "I can't do
spring," she said. "I'm working." Already a decision point. I
could have told God, "See—I'm stuck." Instead by a grace that
surely he provided, I said, "I can't either. I'll call. They'll get
somebody."*

*I called while I still had the momentum, and I made
other calls to re-organize my life, all the while resentful, angry.
I told God that surely I had given up a lot for Lent. The anxiety
raged all through the night, all through the following day, all
through the Holy Thursday Mass.*

*Following the mass, at the Eucharistic Benediction,
something in me let go. Candles gave a rich glow to the chapel.
Kneelers were arranged in circular rows. Before me was the
host, the Body of Jesus, and he loved me. All the crummy feelings*

fell away. I felt pure joy. "Yes, Lord."

I've subsequently said, "Maybe, Lord," and "Not now, Lord," and even possibly, "You've got to be kidding," but the relationship had opened to new dimensions wherein responding to the Lord was one of the dynamics. This conversion experience was healing of soul if not of mind, if the two can be so neatly compartmentalized. I did well for a couple of months and touched base with Fr. Joe from time to time. Toward the end of summer I started to crumble again, and he recommended psychiatric help.

I have occasionally wondered what would have happened if I had skipped the church thing and gone straight to a doc. Healing of the mind is often fraught with upheaval and setback along the way. One feels so alone. I sincerely believe that without that summer hiatus to grow in my relationship with God, the illness would have brought more dire consequences. As it was, there were a few narrow squeaks.

Albeit imperfectly, I gave my life to God. I acknowledge him as my higher power. I don't feel manipulated or controlled. I didn't retire to a cave. In a sense I still feel that I am running my life, but I try to choose God's roads.

I look at my motivations. Is this the right time and place for me to give, or am I looking for the exhilaration of seeing how many balls I can balance in the air at one time? Is it greed? Or a power trip? Or revenge or pettiness? I'll admit that I can easily blind myself to my real motivations, or forget to check them out altogether.

Another question to consider is the possible impact of my choices on those around me. It may or may not be obvious. I might only find out down the road. I sincerely believe that what is truly good for them is good for me. How could it be otherwise?

To me it is important to be on God's roads. There is no guarantee that I will never run out of gas, but I do love him. That's what makes it so important. I still don't know who he is, but we have a relationship.

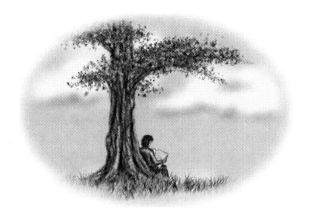

4. The nearness of God.

When something is lost, I tend to look for it in the last place I remember seeing it. If it's not there, I have to look someplace else until I find it. God doesn't get lost, but I can't always find him. That may mean I have to look for him somewhere else.

Scripture.

The Bible is a lovely place to start. What works best for me is to read it daily. Before I had a consistent regimen, I never knew where to turn if I felt a longing for God's word. I had the first few chapters of Genesis pretty well worn out. Although I'll probably never be the type of person who can quote passages, it is possible to build up a repository within oneself to draw upon.

The Old Testament contains three major sections: history, wisdom literature, and prophecy in that order. The history includes many of the familiar stories such as the creation, Abraham, the exodus from Egypt, the conquest of the Promised Land, the succession of kings, the exile to Babylon, and the rebuilding of the Temple. The giving of the commandments to Moses on Mt. Sinai as well as other precepts are in this section, and for that reason it is sometimes called the law.

Job, the first book of the body of wisdom literature, is seen as an allegory rather than a historical event Also included are poetry such as the Psalms, as well as Proverbs and other wisdom literature. The following familiar passage is from the Book of Ecclesiastes:

There is an appointed time for everything,
and a time for every affair under the heavens.
A time to be born, and a time to die;   .
a time to plant, and a time to uproot the plant.
A time to kill, and a time to heal;
a time to tear down, and a time to build.
A time to weep, and a time to laugh;
a time to mourn, and a time to dance.
A time to scatter stones, and a time to gather them;
a time to embrace, and a time to be far from embraces.
A time to seek, and a time to lose;
a time to keep, and a time to cast away.
A time to rend, and a time to sew;
a time to be silent, and a time to speak.
A time to love, and a time to hate;
a time of war, and a time of peace.

Ecclesiastes 3:1-8

The prophets are those who speak for God. This section contains familiar names such as Isaiah and Ezekiel as well as minor prophets like Amos and Habbakuk.

Although spoken to God's people of the time, these passages also contain foreshadowings of the Messiah:

> Therefore the Lord himself shall give you this sign: the virgin shall be with child, and bear a son, and shall name him Immanuel.

Isaiah 7:14

The New Testament begins with the four Gospels—Matthew, Mark, Luke, and John—which tell the Good News, the story of Jesus' time on earth. They are the heart of Scripture, and I spend more time with them than anywhere else. They are followed by the Acts of the Apostles which tell how Jesus' message spread, focusing primarily on Peter and Paul. The epistles are letters written by Paul and others to the new churches and a few individuals to encourage them in their new faith. Finally Revelations is the last book of the Bible, an apocalyptic vision written with a symbolism that has been subject to wide interpretation. Through it we gain a sense of the heavenly Kingdom.

Aids in understanding the Bible include commentaries, Bible dictionaries, concordances, Bible atlases. Some of these I have picked up used, and they are all on my CD-ROM (NIV) Bible. Other inspiring works are meditations such as Merton, lives of saints and writings of saints, and histories of the faith. Many shelves at both religious and secular bookstores are filled with inspirational works. A real blessing is to find a Bible study group or reflection group.

Interacting with God.

There are so many ways to pray, and it seems I've used many of them at one time or another, depending on my needs at the time—short prayers, written prayers, spontaneous prayers, prayers of words, prayers of silence. We communicate "with" God, not just "to" God. It is dialogue, an interactive process. It may not seem that God is participating. If I look out my window as I pray, the clouds don't suddenly form a big "YES." (Or a big "NO.") I usually get a feeling of "Well, okay, then." I'm not sure how God defines "okay," but everything is going to be okay.

Some of the forms of prayers in the Psalms include:
- petition
- thanksgiving
- praise
- repentance

Petition. To petition is to ask for something. We pray for the needs of others, those who are sick or bereaved or lonely or have special needs. We ask God to bless our loved ones. We pray for abstracts such as world peace and racial harmony.

We also pray for ourselves, for healing of body and mind and heart and soul. Some people grew up with the idea that it was selfish and wrong to pray for oneself. I see it as important. Otherwise we would be trying to hold back a piece of ourselves from God by not telling him what we want in our hearts. So many of my prayers start with, "Oh, Lord," as I tell him my frustrations and anxieties.

One-third of the psalms are prayers of individual petition, people asking to be delivered from enemies or illness or even death. Almost all of these end in some expression of confidence wherein the petitioner expresses trust that God has heard. Some examples:

> Do not cast me aside in my old age;
> as my strength fails, do not forsake me,. . .

And the expression of confidence:

> I will always hope in you
> and add to all your praise.

Psalm 71:9, 14

Another example:

> Listen, God, to my prayer;
> do not hide from my pleading;
> hear me and give answer.

And the expression of confidence:

> God will give me freedom and peace
> from those who war against me,
> though there are many who oppose me.

Psalm 55:2-3a, 19

There are many more such examples of a change in mood, a lifting of spirit. Some say these petitions were prayers presented at the temple, and that the upturn was part of the ritualistic formula. Whatever the purpose, it is a very effective way of praying. It helps so much to end a prayer of petition by saying, "I believe you have heard me."

And God hears. Scripture provides countless examples of God listening to the prayers and pleas of his people. One of the most notable is the agony in the garden, when Jesus prayed to God just before his arrest. As Luke tells it,

> After withdrawing about a stone's throw from them [the disciples] and kneeling, he prayed, saying, "Father, if you are willing, take this cup away from me; still, not my will but yours be done." And to strengthen him an angel from heaven appeared to him.
>
> Luke 22:41-43

In this case God's answer to his Son, his beloved One, was strength—a strength so tangible that it took an angel to transport it from heaven.

Or consider when God spoke to Moses from the burning bush:

> "I have witnessed the affliction of my people in Egypt and have heard their cry of complaint against their slave drivers, so I know well what they are suffering."
>
> Exodus 3:7

He went on to say that he would rescue them from the hands of the Egyptians and lead them to a land of milk and honey. He had heard their cry.

Thy will be done. The words are familiar from the Our Father and from Jesus' prayer in the Garden. It is at the heart of every prayer of petition—acceptance of God's will. What he wants is for us to love him, and for us to know that he loves us. Prayer is part of this dialogue of the revelation of God's love.

I also add simple complaint to the heading of prayers of petition, venting to God, as for example in the prayer of Jeremiah who prophesied prior to and during the siege of Jerusalem:

> You duped me, O LORD, and I let myself be duped;
> you were too strong for me, and you triumphed.
> All the day I am an object of laughter;
> everyone mocks me.

> Jeremiah 20:7

Moses was so exasperated by his people that he prayed for death:

> "Why do you treat your servant so badly?" Moses asked the Lord. "Why are you so displeased with me that you burden me with all this people?... I cannot carry all this people by myself, for they are too heavy for me. If this is the way you will deal with me, then please do me the favor of killing me at once, so that I need no longer face this distress."

> Numbers 11:11,14-15

God responded by appointing seventy elders to share the burden of the people with him. A natural inference from this is to realize that suicide is never God's will. Each of us has a life-death switch. Only God's hand belongs on that switch, not ours. Moses was not contemplating suicide. He realized that pulling the switch was God's prerogative.

Thanksgiving. If I can't find God when I look ahead, then I can try to look back. If I acknowledge and give thanks to God for his help in one situation, I tend to remember and feel more confident the next time I need help.

Since my depression, doing the routine became difficult, and doing the difficult has become impossible. That gives me many opportunities to give thanks. I am grateful when I get my laundry done, and I credit it to God. If I ever finish this book, it will be an answer to prayer. Thanks be to God!

> You are my God, and I give you thanks;
> my God, I offer you praise.
> Give thanks to the LORD, for he is good;
> whose love endures forever.

Psalm 118:28-29

Praise. While thanksgiving is often for a specific deed of the Lord ("I was hard pressed and falling, but the LORD came to my help" [Psalm 118:13]), praise is a more generalized recognition of the greatness and goodness of God. The two are closely related, and it is sometimes splitting hairs to try to categorize between them.

God doesn't need praise. He is sufficient unto himself. We need to praise him. We need that sense of awe. As a sentence said only with our heads, "Give glory to God" is pretty ridiculous. Who are we to give him glory? He is glory. On the other hand, as an expression of faith, a cry of exultation, "Give glory to God!" stirs us, puts us however briefly on the borders of the Kingdom to come.

> Sing to the LORD a new song;
>> sing to the LORD, all the earth.
> Sing to the LORD, bless his name;
>> announce his salvation day after day.
>>> Psalm 96:1-2

Other ways to pray.

We communicate with each other in words, both in what we say and how we say it. We also use facial expression, body language, and other forms of nonverbal communication. When we are apart, we can reach out to each other by telephone, letter, email, fax, and FTD florist. We have as many ways of communicating with God, also verbal and nonverbal.

Letters to God. Every now and then I write God in a notebook, but I tear it out and throw it away when finished. It is for God's eyes only. It is an act of saying, "I know that you heard." Journalizing can also take the form of a letter to God.

Music. Christian stores carry tapes or CDs of gospel music, modern liturgical, or other sacred music. Most cities have a radio station devoted to gospel or other religious music. Music is an invitation to God's Kingdom. They say that sung prayer is prayer prayed twice.

Familiar prayers. Many prayers have been passed down through centuries. The most widely known is the Our Father (or Lord's Prayer), which Jesus himself gave us (Matthew 6:9-13; see also Luke 11:2-4].

Other popular prayers are the Hail Mary, or the prayer of St. Francis ("Lord, make me an instrument of your peace...."). Their very familiarity can be a comfort when stressed. Or we may pray the rosary, alone or in groups. Also there are litanies, in which a leader will say, e.g., the name of a saint, and the people will respond, "Pray for us." The rhythm of such prayer drums through us, beats out extraneous thoughts, mesmerizes us into a prayerful state.

Formal meditation, while nonverbal, is fairly structured. It often involves a repeated word or phrase and regulated breathing. As one practices this form of prayer on a regular basis, one enters into increasingly advanced stages of meditation. St. Teresa of Avila described these stages in *Interior Castle.*

I find such intensity a bit beyond my levels of concentration, although I would encourage all who are interested to get a book or videotape on the subject and try. Usually a spiritual director is recommended as well.

Without being as formal, it is possible to spend time quietly in the presence of God, especially when one's head is tired. It may be useful to have a religious picture or crucifix to help focus, but it is a prompt to prayer, not the object of prayer.

It's okay if I don't get an immediate spiritual kick as a result of having prayed. It is possible that in the spiritual plane, something happens even when nothing is apparent. When I water my plant, nothing happens. I don't have to jump back out of the way of a sudden growth spurt. If I don't water it, then it dies. Then I realize that something in fact was happening that I couldn't see.

Are "racing thoughts" a part of prayer? One could argue that, if they occur during prayer time, they are our subconscious thoughts coming to the fore to be expressed to God. Others might say they are distraction, background clutter that keeps us from concentrating on prayer. My personal feeling is that it is a question of balance. If I spend large chunks of time with my thoughts racing and calling it prayer, I may be deceiving myself. But if a few stray ideas creep into my prayer time, they may be worth listening to.

One hears about the differences between "active" and "contemplative" as though they were mutually exclusive. A classic example is the incident of the two sisters, Martha and Mary [Luke 10:38-42]. When Jesus comes to visit, Martha bustles about making preparations (active), while Mary sits at his feet (contemplative). Most people show attributes of each, although they may tend more toward one or the other. The truth is somewhere in between, but not necessarily dead center.

The nearness of Jesus.

Jesus was (and is) God among us. He became God made flesh, God tangible. He is the path to God, or as he said, "I am the way and the truth and the life. No one comes to the Father except through me." [John 14:6]

Jesus even looked like us, not a six-winged seraph such as Isaiah encountered but a man of ten fingers and ten toes. He was like us in all things except sin. He showed compassion even toward those who persecuted him:

> "Jerusalem, Jerusalem, you who kill the prophets and stone those sent to you, how many times I yearned to gather your children together as a hen gathers her brood under her wings, but you were unwilling!"

> Luke 13:34

His farewell prayer for his disciples [John 13-17] is filled with love for them, for us, for the world.

> "As the Father loves me, so I also love you. Remain in my love."

> John 15:9

Jesus played with kids and partied with sinners. He knew what it was to be human. We equate human with imperfection. When we are wrong, we excuse ourselves by saying, "I'm only human." Jesus managed to be human without sinfulness.

He displayed understanding to Thomas, who said he would not believe in the resurrection unless he could touch the nail-holes. Jesus said, go ahead. What you need for faith, you will have. Think of how difficult and abstract faith would be were it not for Jesus. And it is through him that we are saved.

Who, though he was in the form of God,
    did not regard equality with God
    something to be grasped.
Rather, he emptied himself,
    taking the form of a slave,
    coming in human likeness;
    and found human in appearance,
    he humbled himself,
    becoming obedient to death,
    even death on a cross.
Because of this, God greatly exalted him
    and bestowed on him the name
    that is above every name,
    that at the name of Jesus
    every knee should bend,
    of those in heaven and on earth and
    under the earth,
    and every tongue confess that
    Jesus Christ is Lord,
    to the glory of God the Father.

Philippians 2:6-10

Many books have been written about Jesus, some about his life, some theological reflections about who he was. Even children's books about Jesus, with their bright pictures and simple message, are inspiring. As John said at the end of his gospel, "There are also many other things that Jesus did, but if these were to be described individually, I do not think the whole world would contain the books that would be written." [John 21:25]

For me, having Jesus in my life is like reading a book (the story of my life) in the presence of a friend. I call him friend because he said I could [John 15:14-15], but he is in fact the Son of God. He was transfigured on the mountain where he talked with Elijah and Moses [Matthew 17: 1-12]. He died on the cross and was raised again. With him is all the power of God. I don't have any other friends like that.

I don't actually experience Jesus in the room with me. ("Sit over here, today, Lord.") It is an attempt to describe the feeling within. When I try to find an analogy for my experience of him, this is the best I can do. I had an English teacher who said that all analogies limp, and it is so true.

Others have their own ways of expressing their faith. I have met so many people of faith both within the mental health system and outside of it, and their experiences are important to my own faith. Just watching the people go up in the communion line, knowing that they believe what I believe—the physical presence of Jesus in the Eucharist—is affirming.

Jesus calls us to respond to him through those who need us. He tells those who will inherit the Kingdom of heaven:

> "For I was hungry and you gave me food, I was thirsty and you gave me drink, a stranger and you welcomed me, naked and you clothed me, ill and you cared for me, in prison and you visited me.... Amen, I say to you, whatever you did for one of these least brothers of mine, you did for me."

> Matthew 25:35-36,40

And we experience Jesus in ourselves. We have been baptized through him. He has given us gifts to offer that not even depression can take away. We are people of grace, people of the promise of the Kingdom yet to come. Jesus said,

> "In my Father's house there are many dwelling places. If there were not, would I have told you that I am going to prepare a place for you? And if I go and prepare a place for you, I will come back again and take you to myself, so that where I am you also may be."

> John 14:2-3

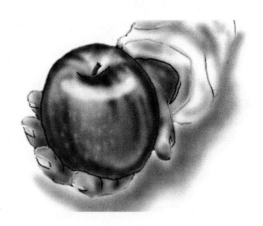

5. What is depression?

Digressing a moment, what is an apple? To a person who is hungry, it is a fruit that tastes good. To a dietitian, it is a source of vitamins A and C. To a juggler, it is red and round. To a grocer, it is a commodity. What something is depends on whom we ask and what type of answer we are seeking.

In the Garden of Eden, when the serpent asked Eve about the fruit tree in the middle of the garden, she saw that "the tree was good for food, pleasing to the eyes, and desirable for gaining wisdom." [Genesis 3:6] Her perception included its function, its appearance, and its benefits.

Similarly there are many ways of defining depression depending on whom we ask.

For those of us who experience depression, it feels like something that has never happened to anyone else ever. It is unique, and we are alone in it.

They tell us that depression is brain chemistry, that our synapses aren't synapsing.

Take two of the purple pills. We are sad because we are sick.

Then they ask us what's been going on in our lives, implying there was some emotional reason for the synapses to stop synapsing. Are we sick because we're sad, or sad because we're sick? It's a bit of chicken-and-egg question, and it is not the intent of this book to resolve it. Recovery lies in breaking out of the cycle.

Physiological framework.

The physiological origin of depression lies in the transmission of impulses along neurons or nerve cells. The neurons are long in comparison to other cells and carry messages in the form of electrical impulses along their membranes. At the end of the neuron is a gap or synapse between it and the next neurons. In order for the message to be transmitted from one neuron to another, the proper substances or neurotransmitters must be present in the synapse in a sufficient amount.

Think of two copper wires on a dry paved surface separated by a couple of inches. If an electrical impulse is applied to the far end of one wire, it will not be transmitted to the next. But if there is standing water on the paved surface, the electrical impulse can be carried along. The brain is more like a jumble of telephone wire with many lines intersecting, but the principle is the same.

One particularly crucial neurotransmitter in the brain is serotonin. If it is depleted, the brain will not function at top efficiency. This is why depression is sometimes called a chemical imbalance, and antidepressants work to restore the balance. Why do these chemical imbalances occur in some people and not others?

The causes of depression.

The answers are not all in yet, but there seem to be some strong indications of causative factors for depression:

- Family history is indicated in many cases of depression but not all.
- Loss and grief, especially if there is a lack of support, can be a factor.
- Negative self-esteem and harsh self-judgment can lead to putting oneself under a lot of internal stress.
- External stress and anxiety can lead to depression. Under stress some people get ulcers. Some get heart palpitations. My mind is my weak point.

With such a variety of causes (and the list is not complete), it is not surprising that there is more than one way to treat depression, to be discussed later in this chapter. There are many possible explanations but there is no easy answer to the question of why I am depressed.

Western culture is oriented toward cause-and-effect. Depression cannot be put in a jar and labeled. It is like a tiger. Its teeth are sharp and hurt, yet its fur is soft and seductive, beckoning us to nestle up alongside it. It has dark streaks running through it, and it has a tail that follows wherever it goes.

The experience of depression.

What depression is and what it feels like are two different things. For that matter, no two experiences of depression are quite the same. There are some similar threads running through many of our experiences.

Time is a dragonfly—it is both dragging and flying. By evening I feel totally disconnected from morning of the same day. It is in the distant past.

I might sit in a chair, doing nothing, planning on getting dressed "any minute now" to go to an appointment. My mind goes off on a tangent. I look at the clock and the minute hand has jumped. Already it is almost too late. I'll skip the shower. Before I can get going, the clock has jumped again. Even if I go in my pajamas, there is no way I can make the appointment. I only sat down for a minute, and yet I've been in that chair for forever, and I don't even remember what I was thinking about that was so important.

Depression is pain. Something hurts, and I don't even know what it is. I can't point to it like a cut or a headache. I can't describe it to make another understand. I don't understand. Please, God, let it stop hurting.

> Be gracious to me, Lord, for I am in distress;
>> with grief my eyes are wasted;
>> my soul and my body spent.
> My life is worn out by sorrow,
>> my years by sighing....
>
> Once I said in my anguish,
>> "I am shut out from your sight."
> Yet you heard my plea,
>> when I cried out to you.

Psalm 31:10-11a, 23

Fears and anxieties.

I don't know if I can trust my frontal lobes. They are supposed to help me distinguish what's real and what's not. I can't be sure if they are doing their job. Knowing I have an illness and knowing I am affected by an illness are two different levels of insight. For instance, when I was 4, I knew I was 4. When someone asked my age, I would hold up four fingers by crossing my thumb over my palm. Yet I didn't feel like I was having childish or 4-year-old thoughts. My thoughts came from me. I felt like me. Even now when they say I have this illness, when my thoughts might be out of synch with the rest of the world, I feel like me. I don't feel distorted.

The far right corner of the ceiling is sagging. I know it's not a trick of shadows because I've sat here before and it never sagged before. Evil spirits are pressing on the ceiling from above, trying to break through and enter the room.

If we know we will have these moments, we learn to plan ahead on how to deal with them. More is said on this in the chapter on recovery. It is important not to let thoughts of evil capture our thinking. God is much stronger. God will protect. We focus on him.

You have the LORD for your refuge;
> you have made the Most High your stronghold.
No evil shall befall you,
> no affliction come near your tent.

Psalm 91:9-10

The time of first coming to grips with depression is scary, and the fears are real. Will I be able to continue to function in my role as employee or homemaker or student? Perhaps not, at least for the time being. It's like falling down stairs, reaching out to try to grab a handhold, but everything I reach out for is already gone.

The bad news is that there may be real losses in depression, although not necessarily. The good news is that there is recovery. It doesn't always mean going back to what we were. After all, if I lived in Paris for several months, I wouldn't come back the same. Depression is an experience to put it mildly. There is a forward path leading out of that experience.

The outsider's perception of depression.

Like a watermelon with its thick green rind hiding the fruit, depression doesn't look like what it tastes like. People have a variety of responses to depression. Part of their response depends on how much they understand, but even a head knowledge of the facts of depression does not guarantee understanding of how the illness affects an individual.

When people are judgmental or critical, their lack of perception is their disability. Consider blind Bartimaeus, who sat by the roadside as Jesus was leaving Jericho. Bartimaeus:

> …sat by the roadside begging. On hearing that it was Jesus of Nazareth, he began to cry out and say, "Jesus, Son of David, have pity on me." And many rebuked him, telling him to be silent. But he kept calling out all the more, "Son of David, have pity on me."

> Mark 10:46-48

Note the actions of the crowd. They don't understand what is going on. Perhaps they were embarrassed that this beggar had the audacity to call out to Jesus. This was after all blind Bartimaeus who sat among them every day. We speculate that they may have viewed him with a mixture of affection and disdain, but not with respect for his personhood. In contrast, Jesus heard a person calling to him.

> Jesus stopped and said, "Call him." So they called the blind man, saying to him, "Take courage; get up, he is calling you." He threw aside his cloak, sprang up, and came to Jesus.
>
> Mark 10:49-50

Again those around Bartimaeus appear not to understand him. They assume he will be afraid. It appears to be condescension. Bartimaeus is anything but afraid as he shows by jumping up and going to Jesus. When he threw aside his cloak, was it a sign that he expected to regain his sight and would be able to find it again?

Finally we have the conclusion, when Jesus shows that there is a bond between him and this blind beggar, and that bond is love.

> Jesus said to him in reply, "What do you want me to do for you?" The blind man replied to him, "Master, I want to see." Jesus told him, "Go your way; your faith has saved you." Immediately he received his sight and followed him on the way.
>
> Mark 10:51-52

The people in the story do not appear to be evil or vindictive. They don't understand. We all know that being blind means not being able to see, but how many of us who are sighted can actually relate to that experience? Similarly with depression, we are so disappointed when those close to us don't understand. Like the people in the story, first they tell us to be quiet, then they tell us to get up and go forward.

What others see depends on what they are looking for. Some are looking for the "old" person, our former pre-illness selves, and are disappointed in not finding it. Some are looking for someone to blame, or to pity in a superior sense. As Jesus said to the crowds about John the Baptizer:

> "What did you go out to the desert to see? A reed swayed by the wind? Then what did you go out to see? Someone dressed in fine clothing? Those who wear fine clothing are in royal palaces. Then why did you go out? To see a prophet? Yes, I tell you, and more than a prophet."
>
> Matthew 11:7-9

What is seen depends on who is looking. The sighted are not necessarily able to see.

Treatment.

Once I came to accept the fact that I had an illness, there was the temptation to look for and count the symptoms like counting the spots on measles. I am really sick, aren't I? There are no visible spots; there is no temperature. There is pain, but not the kind I can point to.

Should I go to a doctor for something I can't define? Which doctor? Part of me feared the doctor would say there was nothing wrong. I would feel foolish, and it would mean that I wouldn't get fixed. Ultimately someone else told me I needed a psychiatrist. Before the big break, my milder depressions were diagnosed as things like sinusitis and possible hypoglycemia. I believe GPs have become more aware of the signs of depression and the possible need for referral. There are several treatment options to consider.

Hospitals.

At my second visit, the dragonlady recommended that I go into the hospital for two weeks. All I knew of a hospital was the medical side (specifically maternity) where one lies in bed in a nightgown for a couple of restless days. I knew I was very tired by that point, but I didn't want to spend two weeks in bed. I told her no.

When I finally wound up in the hospital six months later, it was nothing as I had envisioned. People got up and got dressed and got involved in therapeutic settings like groups and activities. As I rose in privilege levels, passes became possible. Most importantly, I met others like myself. I had an illness, not an aberration.

Hospitalization is not indicated for everybody or even most. Insurance considerations are a factor. Legally in most states a person cannot be compelled to stay in a psychiatric hospital or unit involuntarily beyond an evaluation period unless she has been found in a court hearing to be dangerous to herself or others.

I would have done better to enter the hospital when it was first recommended. Finding the right psychotropic meds would have been easier and safer, and my family and

I would have been spared a lot of pain. In the intervening six months, I only got sicker. I wound up spending two months instead of two weeks and was on my third doctor by then.

I went through phases in my hospitalizations. For the first few times, I was docile as a child, eager to please. After several times I was more like an adolescent when inpatient, rebellious and fighting with staff. The last few times I felt like an adult and calmly asserted my rights, which I had finally learned. The rights guaranteed by law are not necessarily the same as the rights posted on the bulletin board or handed to me at intake. I also learned that each state has a Protection & Advocacy agency for the protection of the rights of people with mental illness.

Medications.

Medications are not a magic bullet, pop two of the blue and four of the red and everything will be fine. It is an inexact science. It may take time to find the right med or combination. Even when the blood level of the medications is right on target, it is possible to crash and land in the hospital. Meds help many people. It is a question to consider carefully.

Knowledge is the key. I know what I am taking, what it's for, and the possible side effects. I pretty much know what I have taken at other times, especially what didn't work. It might have been useful to keep a log.

There are several important sources for more information on a medication:

> • my doctor,
> • the Physician's Desk Reference, available at the library,

- the Internet, especially the sites of the pharmaceutical companies,
- the pharmacist.

There are those who feel one is not "recovered" from mental illness unless one is off medications. I don't agree. I look at the possibility that I may have to take medications for the rest of my life. That doesn't bother me. What matters is trying to be part of a world with other people, caring about them in that world, operating with some degree of functionality in that world. By working with my doctor, I have reduced my level of medication to some degree.

I have met people in the hospital who went off their meds. One woman told me she had felt better and had stopped taking them. Within four months she was sick again. I have met other people with other reasons for rebelling against the meds. I also have friends who have gone off their medications in consultation with their doctors, tapering down carefully, and watching for positive and negative effects.

Psychotherapy.

Therapy is a term that is used loosely. It can mean something that is good for me, for example, a walk is therapeutic. It can refer to certain types of groups in hospitals or day programs, such as art therapy. Probably we most commonly think of one-on-one sessions with a psychiatrist, a therapist, or a counselor. Therapists often have degrees such as LPCC or LISW or Psy.D. They may belong to professional organizations. Some states have few if any regulations about who can hang out a shingle as therapist or counselor. A psychiatrist is an M.D. and is able to prescribe medications.

Some maintain there are over 200 types of psychotherapy, from Freudian analysis to primal scream. To confuse matters more, many therapists do not adhere strictly to one school of thought but draw from the ideas of several.

For me the first visit with a psychiatrist or therapist has usually been pretty easy. It's a matter of taking history, answering general questions. The second session has been less directed, and I've floundered. Most often something has clicked by the sixth visit. If not, I've moved on.

I left the one I called the dragonlady after six weeks. I also left quickly the one who felt he should repeat part of our discussions to my husband. One psychiatrist had a practice in her basement. I entered through the garage. Her desk was piled 6 inches in papers with a couple of shoe boxes of drug samples on top. She rattled one shoe box at me and asked me what I wanted to take. Nothing, thank you. I didn't go back.

Even a few very nice people made me feel like I wasn't getting anywhere in trying to talk to them. I had a friend who said his therapist never spoke, just grunted, and that his dog was more intelligent. To change therapists constantly might be a sign of avoidance of the process. I've felt some were helping me get better. One I left when I moved out of state, and another because of insurance reasons. I've been with my current doctor for several years.

Holistic medicine.

Out of curiosity, I entered the word "holistic" on a search engine on the Internet. I was rewarded with 1.4 million hits, or web sites. Some were from serious organizations devoted to the practice of holistic medicine. Some were quite frankly people who had something to sell, who were capitalizing on a word that has become popular.

One definition given for holistic medicine is the following:

> Holistic medicine is a system of health care which fosters a cooperative relationship among all those involved, leading towards optimal attainment of the physical, mental, emotional, social and spiritual aspects of health. It emphasizes the need to look at the whole person, including analysis of physical, nutritional, environmental, emotional, social, spiritual and lifestyle values. It encompasses all stated modalities of diagnosis and treatment including drugs and surgery if no safe alternative exists. Holistic medicine focuses on education and responsibility for personal efforts to achieve balance and well being.
>
> Canadian Holistic Medical Association

Some describe it as an alternative to traditional medicine. I'm not sure of the need to choose between one or the other. Perhaps the truth is somewhere in between. It would seem that it would be feasible for holistic techniques to be used in conjunction with traditional therapies and medications. If God had only one answer for every question, then all flowers would be red.

Exactly what is included in holistic practice varies from list to list. The focus in the definition above is on education and personal responsibility. I offer below a partial list of additional forms of therapy/treatment which can be used. Some would be considered holistic.

- movement—exercise, dance, walking, swimming
- tae bo, tai chi, yoga
- arts—art therapy, music therapy, etc.
- massage
- aromatherapy
- meditation—including prayer
- journalizing, writing
- acupuncture, acupressure

Many of the above are usually solitary or conducted with a therapist in that discipline. Socialization is a form of healing, whether in a support group or volunteer group or church group or a couple of close friends.

Mind-set.

One often-overlooked part of any treatment is our attitude toward healing. We have to be ready to pray, "Lord, I want to heal." In the beginning of Matthew 8, a leper came to Jesus and said, "Lord, if you will to do so, you can cure me." Jesus touched him and said, "I do will it. Be cured." Immediately the man was cured. Jesus wills it, but do we want to be healed? Are we willing to approach him with that request?

There are reasons why we are reluctant to heal, in spite of the obvious advantages.

Some of the more common reasons:

- I have finally found a safe and stable place for myself within the depression. I don't want to rock the boat.
- I am afraid that there will be nothing there when I emerge.

• I don't want to face the debris, such as ruptured relationships, that was created when I was sick.

If these and other reluctances arise during reflective moments, we can counter them with the simple prayer, "Lord, I want to heal." We are taking the leap into faith.

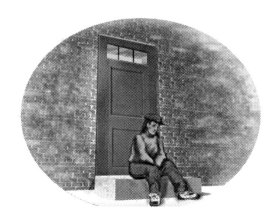

6. Why me?

In our human (and limited) concept of justice, God rewards the good and punishes the wicked. Scripture does speak at times of God's anger. What is that about? The concepts of good and evil, reward and punishment, can be seen in Moses' last words to the Israelites.

> "Here, then, I have today set before you life and prosperity, death and doom. If you obey the commandments of the LORD, your God, which I enjoin on you today, loving him, and walking in his ways, and keeping his commandments, statutes, and decrees, you will live and grow numerous, and the LORD, your God, will bless you in the land you are now entering to occupy. If, however, you turn away your hearts and will not listen, but are led astray and adore and serve other gods, I tell you now that you will certainly perish; you will not have a long life on the land which you are crossing the Jordan to enter and occupy. I call heaven and earth today to witness against you; I have set before you life and death, the blessing and the curse."

Deuteronomy 30:15-19

The last section of the Old Testament is devoted to the writing of the prophets. These were men that God called to speak for him, such as Isaiah, Jeremiah, Ezekiel, and others. It is worth noting that, on being called to prophesy, many of them asked, "Why me?" The people at the time of the writings of the prophets had strayed from worship of the one true God. They cheated in business, cheated in marriage (including bringing prostitutes into the temple for pagan fertility rites) and even sacrificed their own children to false gods. The prophets tried to warn Israel and Judah to return to God. They said that the Lord was angry and would bring upon the people famine, pestilence, and sword, but they also spoke of the promise of restoration of the nation when they returned to God. The curse and the blessing. Either way, the language strikes resonant chords within us.

> Therefore, thus says the Holy One of Israel:
>> Because you reject this word,
> And put your trust in what is crooked and devious,
>> and depend on it,
> This guilt of yours shall be
>> like a descending rift
> Bulging out in a high wall
>> whose crash comes suddenly, in an instant....
>
> Yet the LORD is waiting to show you favor,
>> and he rises to pity you;
> For the LORD is a God of justice:
>> blessed are all who wait for him!
>
> O people of Zion who dwell in Jerusalem,
>> no more will you weep;

He will be gracious to you when you cry out,
>> as soon as he hears he will answer you.

Isaiah 30:12-13, 18-20

Is depression a manifestation of the wrath of God? Is God that angry? Have I been that bad? I know I haven't been saintly, but this is awful. And if God Almighty is angry, where do I turn for help?

In the Old Testament book named after him, Job asked God these questions. He had been an upright, God-fearing man who enjoyed many blessings, but he was then afflicted horribly. In a series of mishaps he lost his herds (his wealth), his grown sons and daughters, and his health. Covered with painful boils and open sores, he went to sit on the heap of ashes outside of the city to mourn. Why me, Lord? What have I done?

Three friends came to support Job. Friends haven't changed over the years. There are always some who mean well but have it all wrong. In a cycle of speeches they suggested to Job that he was being punished for his sins. Eliphaz said,

>> "Reflect now, what innocent person perishes?
>> Since when are the upright destroyed?"

Job 4:7

Job pleaded his innocence.

>> "Teach me, and I will be silent;
>> prove to me wherein I have erred.

Job 6:24

61

Job challenged God:

> "I will say to God: Do not put me in the wrong!
> > Let me know why you oppose me.
> Is it a pleasure for you to oppress,
> > to spurn the work of your hands,
> > and smile on the plan of the wicked?"

Job 10:2-3

Job complained to God:

> "Why then did you bring me forth from the womb?
> > I should have died and no eye have seen me.
> I should be as though I had never lived;
> > I should have been taken from the womb to the grave."

Job 10: 18-19

How many of us in our depression have wished we had never been born? Job is the Everyman who suffers for no apparent reason. For no cause that he could discern, he seemed to have lost favor with God. He was experiencing not just the loss of property or of family or of health, but also the loss of the vital God-relationship. Why me, Lord? What have I done that you would turn from me?

The dialogues with the friends continued. A fourth man named Elihu appeared. After all had their say, God addressed Job out of the storm. Essentially, his answer was, "Hang on a minute here. Which of us is God?"

> "Who is this that obscures divine plans
> > with words of ignorance?

Gird up your loins now, like a man;
I will question you, and you tell me the answers!
Where were you when I founded the earth?
Tell me, if you have understanding.
Who determined its size; do you know?
Who stretched out the measuring line for it?
Into what were its pedestals sunk,
and who laid the cornerstone,
While the morning stars sang in chorus
and all the sons of God shouted for joy?

Job 38:2-7

God is playful, as a parent ruffling the hair of an unhappy child, as he describes (in chapters 39 and 40) some of the more inventive of his creations:

"Do you know about the birth of the mountain goats?" [39:1]
"Will the wild ox consent to serve you?" [39:9]
"Is it by your discernment that the hawk soars?" [39:26]
"Can you lead about Leviathan [maybe crocodile] with a hook?" [40:25]

Job conceded the point and repented for challenging God. Only God is God, and his ways are inscrutable. We can question the wisdom of God, but we won't necessarily understand the answer, because God's wisdom is so far above us.

Why Job?

Even though we can't know God's reasons, we still search for one, and in this instance we are given the context at the beginning of the story. Remember that this is an allegory, a story with a message, rather than a true account. In the Bible, the Book of Job is with the wisdom literature rather than with the history.

In chapter 1, God asked the satan if he'd noticed Job, who was blameless and upright, who feared God and avoided evil. (A commentary suggests that "the satan" should be taken to mean "the Adversary" rather than the devil as the term was used later in Scripture.) The satan replied that it was for good reason that Job was God-fearing. After all, God had blessed Job and all he had. But if God were to take those blessings away, the satan was sure that Job would blaspheme God.

God gave the satan permission to bring misfortune to Job. The series of calamities began. Job complained and challenged God, but he never blasphemed God. He remained a God-fearing man.

I have blasphemed God. It's not the same as being angry. It was writing him off in my heart, rejecting that commitment to follow him. I don't even remember what upset me so much. That's how trivial it must have been in perspective. I do remember writing him off, with the f-word at that.

The next morning at mass, everything went wrong. I went because my son was an altar-server. One of the candles wouldn't stay lit. We started the mass with one candle. During the eucharistic prayer, a fat and ugly August fly crawled around the side of the altar cloth toward me. It was an early mass, but already the heat was building up in the bowl-shaped chapel. The other altar-server, a bigger, beefy kid in early adolescence, passed out as they kneeled at the side of the altar. His parents revived him and got him out of there.

I don't believe that, in a mass for two hundred people, God arranged these "signs" just for me. I believe that the things that my heart noticed were God's way of speaking to me. Maybe somebody else noticed the flowers. That may have been how God spoke to them that morning. I don't remember if there were flowers. I have no idea what the Gospel or homily was about. Perhaps they struck someone else's heart. Maybe the kid had skipped breakfast. Adolescents are like that.

Whatever it was, it chilled my heart. I haven't since put aside the Lord in the same way. I still think it might be okay to get angry with him, telling him what's bugging me to his face, but not turning my back. I don't find myself angry as often either. I understand something better now. I don't understand what it is that I understand, but I understand. It's about trust.

Things happen. Stuff happens, to paraphrase a bumper sticker. The world is flawed. It can be a problem perpetrated by humankind, or a breakdown in our own bodies or minds, or an act of nature. If a tornado rips through a church and pulls off the roof, is that a sign from God that the church was bad? When Job suffered, was it because of sin? God's answer is that we cannot read the mind of God. He is too vast. Only he knows whether it was the chicken or the egg. I take comfort in knowing that he loves us and cares about what happens to us:

> We know that all things work for good for those who love God, who are called according to his purpose.

> Romans 8:28

I remember a dark time of doubt and despair and anxiety, when it seemed that God had set things up so I would surely fail.

The God of the Low Places

I happened to have coffee with a homeless man whom I had met after weekday mass. We were discussing theology generally. "Pray with conviction," the man said "When you pray, you must pray with conviction."

The proverbial scales fell from my eyes. Suddenly I could see that I was going to make it through the tough times, that things were going to be okay, and they were. They even felt okay.

It is not the only time that God has reached out with love and used another to touch me when I was seriously doubting or turned away. He does not always chastise. Sometimes when we love our neighbors, it turns out that God sent them.

Whatever the situation, God can turn it to good. St. Paul (who wrote the above passage) was a New Testament person who suffered precisely because he was doing good in his efforts to spread the Gospel. In the following passage, he uses his suffering to prove that he is dedicated to the churches to which he ministered, in contrast to false ministers.

Five times at the hands of the Jews I received forty lashes minus one. Three times I was beaten with rods, once I was stoned, three times I was shipwrecked, I passed a night and a day on the deep; on frequent journeys, in dangers from rivers, dangers from robbers, dangers from my own race, dangers from Gentiles; dangers in the city, dangers in the wilderness, dangers at sea, dangers among false brothers; in toil and hardship, through many sleepless nights; through hunger and thirst, through frequent fastings, through cold and exposure. And apart from these things, there is the daily pressure upon me of my anxiety for all the churches.

2 Corinthians 11:24-28

I don't like suffering any more than anyone else. I don't volunteer for it. I don't self-inflict. Neither did Paul, but he knew that his very suffering was a sign that he was with God. When I feel pain for someone who is suffering, it means that I am human, and to be human is the path to the divine.

God uses us, as he used Paul, as he used the homeless man. Recovered alcoholics give leads at meetings and sponsor new members to help in their recovery. People recovering from mental illness get involved in consumer movements for the benefit of other consumers. Whatever the form of suffering, it is those who have gone before who offer most hope and encouragement to the newly afflicted.

In instructing his apostles, Jesus said,

"When you have done all you have been commanded, say, 'We are unprofitable servants; we have done what we were obliged to do.'"

Luke 17:10

Was it my fault?

When I ask, "Why me?" inevitably my thoughts drift to the further question, "Is this my fault? Is this some subconscious game on my part?" Certainly enough people have told me to snap out of it as if it were within my power to do so. I can remember how encouraged I was when I read Psalm 103:

> Bless the LORD, my soul;
>> and all my being, bless his holy name!
> Bless the LORD, my soul,
>> do not forget all the gifts of God,
> Who pardons all your sins,
>> heals all your ills,
> Delivers your life from the pit,
>> surrounds you with love and compassion,
> Fills your days with good things;
>> your youth is renewed like the eagle's.

> Psalm 103:1-5

God forgives sins and heals diseases. It doesn't matter what we label it. He can deal with it. It's like calling AAA in the winter and saying, "Maybe it's the carburetor. Or maybe I didn't winterize the radiator." AAA doesn't care. They send a truck which tows it to a mechanic to be fixed. It's that easy. It doesn't matter. Our youth will be renewed like an eagle's.

Guilt can be useful, as when our conscience tells us we have done something wrong. On the other hand, our sense of guilt can be over-active. When we are hurting, when we are suffering, we tend to assume it is all our fault, even though we are not sure what we have done to deserve all this. St. Teresa of Avila described some of the suffering of depression, and went on to say:

> There are occasions when one cannot help doing this [letting thoughts wander]: times of ill-health (especially in persons who suffer from melancholia); or times

when our heads are tired, and, however hard we try, we cannot concentrate; or times when, for their own good, God allows His servants for days on end to go through great storms.... The very suffering of anyone in this state will show her that she is not to blame, and she must not worry, for that only makes matters worse, nor must she weary herself by trying to put sense into something—namely, her mind—which for the moment is without any.[3]

We need to lighten up on ourselves. The suffering we are experiencing is not punishment for something we have done. Most of us have at some time experienced someone saying, "Shame on you" (or an equivalent) and wagging a finger in our faces. Because of these deep experiences, shame is one of the most painful feelings we deal with. What a sense of relief it was to discover that depression is a shame-free, guilt-free illness. The Lord rules.

+ Mistakes can make us feel guilty. I remember thinking with remorse that if I had sought help earlier in my illness, I wouldn't have needed to get so sick. That may have been true, but it was a mistake, not a sin. Remorse happens when we don't let go of our feelings of wrongness and guilt, don't offer our muddiness to Jesus to + be cleaned.

+ As we grow more confident in God's love and forgiveness, we don't even need to split hairs. Maybe it was pride that kept me from seeking help. Maybe I just didn't have the information I needed. What has happened, has happened. I can't make it unhappen. I am sorry for my responsibility in it. I look forward to how God will bring good out of it.

Why me?

Early in my illness, I asked God, why me? Sometimes I felt his answer was, "It had to be somebody. I knew you could handle it." My illness then seemed like a compliment from the Lord. That alone is a usefulness—to take up our share of the suffering of the world. Nobody promised we would be without burdens. The fact that something happens to someone does not mean that it was a punishment for sin. Jesus taught the same lesson in the New Testament:

> "Or those eighteen people who were killed when the tower at Siloam fell on them—do you think they were more guilty than everyone else who lived in Jerusalem? By no means!"

Luke 13:4-5a

In today's terms, we might ask if the thousands who died when the World Trade Center towers collapsed were somehow more sinful than other people. Certainly not! They were the innocent victims of evil.

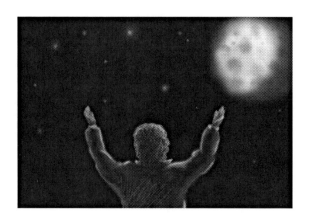

7. Who are we?

Like the mathematical equation $x = y$, there are two sides to the God-relationship. It is not enough to have a concept of God. We also have to know who we are. Why did he create us? Do we each have value individually as persons?

If nothing else, I am human, a biped, a primate, an animal like other animals with a few important exceptions. We say, "I'm only human," when we admit our frailties, but in fact to be human is to be at the pinnacle of God's creation on earth.

> When I see your heavens, the work of your fingers,
> > the moon and the stars that you set in place
> What are humans that you are mindful of them,
> > mere mortals that you care for them?
> Yet you have made them little less than a god,
> > crowned them with glory and honor.
> You have given them rule over the works of your hands,
> > put all things at their feet.

Psalm 8:4-7

Other species evolve. Birds learn to make nests. It becomes patterned in their brains over centuries. Human beings progress. They read blueprints and study engineering. They learn how to make cathedrals and skyscrapers. The thoughts of those who lived before us are available to us. Humans are able to compound and build on information from one generation to the next in an exponential stream of technological growth.

Who am I to me? What do we know about ourselves individually? We hold weight and take up space—we have bodies. As Descartes said, I think; therefore I am. We have minds. We know we have hearts, metaphysical seats of emotionality, because we have felt them in both joy and pain. We are creations of the breath of God. We have souls. Body, mind, heart, soul—the neat yet overlapping categories by which we sum up our human existence. They impact on each other. If I am out Christmas shopping and my bunion hurts, I feel less giving in my heart, more exasperated in my mind, less in touch with the reason for the season in my soul.

Our soul is what distinguishes us from other animals, but much of what we consider soul is reposed in the mind (as opposed to physical brain). This is what makes a mind a terrible thing to lose. Consider what happened to the once powerful King Nebuchadnezzar of Babylon, who earlier conquered Jerusalem and carried her inhabitants off into exile:

> Nebuchadnezzar was cast out from among men, he ate grass like an ox, and his body was bathed with the dew of heaven, until his hair grew like the feathers of an eagle, and his nails like the claws of a bird.

> Daniel 4:30

If having a mind distinguishes us from animals, then to lose one's mind threatens our very sense of humanity. Even if we don't often exhibit signs of psychosis or delusion, our minds feel fragile, and we are definitely having a problem getting them to function. It is the only illness that strikes at our core concept of being human. We are afraid we will wind up as an animal like Nebuchadnezzar.

Often mental illness is depicted in the Bible as demonic possession. It reflected the culture of the times. They had very little understanding of the function of the parts of the body. What other conclusions could they have come to? Other cultures have also jumped to the same conclusion. For instance, in Japan, which didn't have any interactions with the Israelites, spirits of the dead were thought to cause demonic possession.

We do feel taken over. Often I feel like I am my mental illness. Period. I have a new label, my diagnosis, a number in *DSM-IV.* Every shred of personality I had before my illness seems to have been blown away. I feel less articulate. I weigh more, and I look dumpy. I am a walking depressed area, a bubblehead who can't remember anything. I have become absorbed in the illness.

Depression is a time when self-esteem is low, both cause and effect in a vicious circle: we are down on ourselves because we feel we are not fulfilling our roles in life, and we are depressed because we are down on ourselves.

We let go of how others look at us. To paraphrase the Serenity Prayer, some of the mud I see in myself I can shovel away, some of the mud I must walk through, and the trick is to know the difference. What of myself do I accept? What of myself can I change? And what do I despair of?

Am I disabled?

The synonyms in my thesaurus for disability are just awful. They include incapacity, inability, unfitness, helplessness, powerlessness, weakness. It seems so unfair. I often feel that the persons coping with a disability are stronger than those who are more able. For instance, the woman who comes to church using a walker, who clumps down the aisle pausing at each step while her back foot catches up with the rest of her, shows more persistence, more dedication, more strength than those of us who shuffled in on two good limbs. Moreover she smiles on her way in. That's the real test of strength.

To be eligible for Social Security Disability Insurance (SSDI) or Supplemental Security Income (SSI), one must meet their definition of disability:

> We consider you disabled under Social Security rules if you cannot do work that you did before and we decide that you cannot adjust to other work because of your medical condition(s).

www.ssa.gov

Often our job titles are how we define ourselves, especially to others, and with disability that job title is taken away.

Conversation with a woman from church:
Her: What do you do?
Me: I do what I can.

Her: I'd go crazy if I didn't work.

The Equal Employment Opportunities Commission uses a functional definition for determining who is eligible for protection under the Americans with Disabilities Act. Eligibility does not depend on diagnosis but what major life activities a person can perform.

> The major life activities limited by mental impairments differ from person to person. There is no exhaustive list of major life activities. For some people, mental impairments restrict major life activities such as learning, thinking, concentrating, interacting with others, caring for oneself, speaking, performing manual tasks, or working. Sleeping is also a major life activity that may be limited by mental impairments.
>
> EEOC Enforcement Guidance on the ADA and Psychiatric Disabilities

There are people truly deserving of these benefits and protections by law, but it means wearing the label "disabled." Unfortunately our self-concept is affected by the labels we wear. Consider this scene from an unpublished novel. Nan is Shirley's daughter. Shirley had hurt her back a year earlier in an automobile accident and needs a wheelchair.

> After wiping the table, Nan brought out the three thin boxes containing the gift certificates and proceeded to wrap them. One end of the second box looked lumpy, and she taped it down impatiently.
> "It's only flimsy paper," Shirley commented from her spectator position on the side of the table.

"You're stronger than it. Make it do what you want it to."

"Perhaps there's something on television," Nan said, searching under the scraps of paper for the pen to write the gift tag.

"If you disciplined yourself to put the pen in the same place every time, you'd always have it."

"Is there more tape?"

"Put it on the shopping list. One roll should have been enough."

"It was mostly gone when I started." Nan tossed the empty tape dispenser onto the scraps of paper. "I don't see why I'm doing this. You're not an invalid."

"I am too an invalid." Shirley sat immobile while Nan glared at her. Nan shook her head and rose from the table, returned with coat in hand. "I meant that you are just as capable as I to sit at the table and wrap packages. More capable to hear you tell it. I'm beginning to think I'm the invalid for letting you do this to me."

Chicken Anger, unpublished

When someone suggests we might not be all that disabled, we want to shout back, "I am too disabled." We are afraid that they will expect of us more than we can give. Disabled comes to mean "can't do"—can't cook, can't clean, can't shop, can't shower, can't read, can't sleep, can't walk, can't work. It is self-limiting. Of the eight can't-do things on the above list (which is not exhaustive), I have three currently. I've had more in the past.

We are like the sick man at the Sheep Pool in Bethesda (see John 5:1-9). Legend had it that when the waters were stirred up, the first one into the pool would be healed. Many blind, lame, infirm were waiting at the pool for the waters to be stirred up. Because of his disability, this particular man was never able to get to the pool quickly enough.

When Jesus came and asked why he was there, he replied that he had no one to carry him to the water when it was stirred up. Perhaps he was hoping that Jesus would carry him. Instead, Jesus told him to take up his mat and walk.

The man had a big "can't do," namely, getting to the water, and yet he stayed at the pool. He obviously hoped that some good would come of being in the right place, and it did.

That is a way to treat our own disabilities, our "can't-do" items. Rather than crossing them off the list for all time, we can stay in the can-do zone, stay in the right place to resume them when we are ready.

For some time I could only concentrate on a paragraph at a time before I got distracted by my own thoughts. Nevertheless I would pick up things that looked interesting and get a little further. At first it was mostly The Sporting News, relatively short articles, easy to follow, and I was interested in sports. Now I enjoy reading whole books, especially fiction. I keep a running list of the names of characters and the page they first appeared to help me keep them straight.

Cooking is something I don't do. It is hard to remember to add all the ingredients, or even to remember that there is something on the stove, and it seems pointless for one person. So many foods go from freezer to microwave. It's easy to get out of practice. To stay in the can-do zone I occasionally bake something for the people at work. They are always hungry. If we hang around the right place long enough, God will be there.

> Then the LORD said [to Elijah], "Go outside and stand on the mountain before the LORD; the LORD will be passing by." A strong and heavy wind was rending the mountains and crushing rocks before the LORD —but the LORD was not in the wind. After the wind there was an earthquake—but the LORD was not in the earthquake. After the earthquake there was fire—but the LORD was not in the fire. After the fire there was a tiny whispering sound. When he heard this, Elijah hid his face in his cloak and went and stood at the entrance of the cave. A voice said to him, "Elijah, why are you here?"

> 1 Kings 19:11-13

Every now and then I get a tiny whispering—this is now possible.

Who am I to others?

I am like a tinsel Christmas tree on which is shining a spotlight with a revolving wheel of colored filters. I am red, now blue, now green, now yellow. Who I am to others depends on what they are looking for, what filter they use. Some see sickness, some stubbornness, some struggle, some love. St. Paul wrote of relating to others:

> To the Jews I became like a Jew to win over Jews; to those under the law I became like one under the law— though I myself am not under the law—to win over those under the law. To those outside the law I became

like one outside the law—though I am not outside God's law but within the law of Christ—to win over those outside the law. To the weak I became weak, to win over the weak. I have become all things to all, to save at least some.

1 Corinthians 9:20-23

Every Wednesday after the day program I picked up the kids from elementary school for our midweek visitation. One week in particular we went to the public library. Tommy went to the children's section to find books, Susie checked to see if there were any Agatha Christie's that she hadn't read, and Mickey did research for a paper. I browsed the stacks. After a while I rounded them up, and we went to my place for supper.

The next day the crafts unit from the day program went to the same library to look for crafts projects for Christmas. The six of us followed along behind as the two staff persons selected books from the shelves. We sat together at the table. As we looked over the books, I asked to go to the restroom. When we had finished, we all went back to the day program together in the van. When I was with the kids, I was the mom. When I was with staff, I was the consumer.

Stigma.

That there is a stigma surrounding mental illness is not news, and depression falls under the umbrella of the stigma as often as not. The stigma comes from fear, prejudice, and superstition. One would think the illness was highly contagious. We are seen as being unpredictable if not dangerous, when in fact the incidence of violence for people with mental illness is almost as small as for the population as a whole.

The question is whether we can come in under the radar, so to speak, to pass for what Fred Friese calls CNPs (chronically normal people). Does it show? Are people saying behind our backs that there's something not quite right about this one? If I go away for a hospitalization, how do I explain it to my employer or the neighbor who took my kid to soccer practice?

It has been said that given a long enough lever and a place to stand, one could move the world. If we try to change the world to accept us, we find we have no place to stand. If we write a television station or newspaper objecting to slurs concerning mental illness (i.e., nutcase, out of his gourd), our letter is dismissed because we are "crazy." I hope that the day will soon come when political correctness is applied to mental illness.

Self-disclosure.

Knowing that there is such a stigma, with each new encounter we have to ask ourselves if we should tell them about our mental illness. What the words mean to us and what the words mean to them are probably very different. Unless they've had experience directly or indirectly, their concept of a psych ward is nothing short of loony bin. (The word bedlam, meaning uproar or confusion, is derived from the popular name for the Hospital of St. Mary of Bethlehem, a London insane asylum.) Mental illness is not the most important thing to know about me, but I don't feel fully accepted if I withhold it. Would they still like me if they knew? At work I don't know who knows I am a consumer or how they found out.

I have been rejected because of mental illness in big ways and small, as most of us have been. I've learned to compromise. I don't tell people when I first meet them, nor at the second or third encounter. When not working, I stayed quiet about my means of support (primarily SSDI). Few people are going to come right out and ask. If we seem to be getting to know each other pretty well, I may confide in them. By then we have some sense of who we are to each other, and knowledge of the diagnosis may not have the same impact.

Part of me feels I am holding back until this particular conversation occurs. I want them to accept all of me. Probably most people who have some closet to come out of feel the same. When Jesus sent his disciples out to teach, he told them,

> "Look for a worthy person in every town or village you come to and stay with him until you leave. As you enter his home bless it. If the home is deserving, your blessing will descend on it. If it is not, your blessing will return to you. If anyone does not receive you or listen to what you have to say, leave that house or town, and once outside it shake its dust from your feet."

Matthew 10:11-14

We know when we've been rejected. Our disclosure comes back to us with a polite "Oh," a throat-clearing, a statement that they currently have all the volunteers they need but will call us as soon as they need us. The phone never rings. When did anybody ever have all the volunteers they needed? It is time to shake the dust from our feet and move on.

Who are we to God?

This is a far easier question. God tells us who we are to him, and his word can be trusted. We are precious in his eyes. Our names are engraved on the palms of his hands [Isaiah 49:15-16]. Jesus said,

> "Are not five sparrows sold for two small coins? Yet not one of them has escaped the notice of God. Even the hairs of your head have all been counted. Do not be afraid. You are worth more than many sparrows."

> Luke 12: 6-7

Aren't sparrows delightful to watch? In watching me, God laughs a lot. I stamp my feet and tell him, "It's not funny. I've been a schmuck again, less than kind, less than loving."

"I know," he answers, "but at least you care about whether you've been kind. It's such a delight to watch you try to love, like watching a toddler try to walk."

Yes, he laughs at me, and I'm glad that he does. It's a comfortable, comforting laugh. And if I lose a hair in the shower, God adjusts the count. His knowledge of me is that intimate, that ongoing.

Then who are we?

If we look harder, we see that much of ourselves is still there, although we are not always able to tap into it. One exercise done in groups is Twenty Questions, not the bigger-than-a-breadbox kind we used to play in the car as kids, but making a list on paper of twenty words that answer the question, "Who am I?" We each answered with whatever nouns or adjectives that came to mind and seemed to fit.

If I were to do that now, my list would include mid-fifties, writer, hopeful, tired. An even more difficult exercise is to use no negative descriptors. Scratch tired. Substitute healthy, thanks be to God. Either way, it's not easy to get to twenty.

Consider how unlikely it is that any two people would have all of the same answers. We are unique; we are individuals each created by God. According to Hasidism,

> It is the duty of every person in Israel to know and consider that he is unique in the world in his particular character and that there has never been anyone like him in the world, for if there had been someone like him, there would have been no need for him to be in the world. Every single man [and woman] is a new thing in the world and is called upon to fulfill his particularity in this world.[4]

We are all miracles. Physically, the DNA of each of us is unique. Also our experiences are unique. Even just for today there is nobody who was in all of the same places at the same times as I. We are children of God.

> You formed my inmost being;
> > you knit me in my mother's womb.
> I praise you, so wonderfully you made me;
> > wonderful are your works!
>
> Psalm 139:13-14

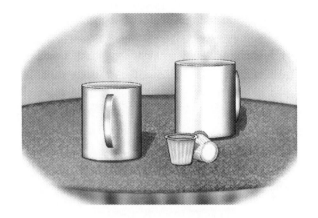

8. Relationships.

Just as we define God in part by our relationship to him, so also we are defined in part by our relationships with others. If each of us is unique, then a relationship is doubly unique, since it involves two (or more) unique individuals.

Mental illness places a huge strain on our relationships. People don't understand what has happened to us or why we don't make it unhappen. Also, we may feel uncomfortable with them, as if we are not part of the same world any more. We have different types of relationships in our lives.

Parents.

Each of us began as an egg from one person and a sperm from another. Some people were raised by those persons, that is, their natural parents. Some were raised by one parent or some other person(s) or even collectively by the staff of an institution. None of us sprang into adulthood on our own. Someone taught us to button our shirts and tie our shoes. We have different experiences of having been raised. Caregivers can be loving or indifferent or abusive or all of the above. Scripture shows us the mother and foster father of Jesus in the beautiful infancy narratives in Matthew and Luke. We also have glimpses of the families of Samuel and David and the sons of Zebedee. Origins are important.

Whether we experienced love as we grew up has a tremendous impact on whether we are naturally able to know and love God. Even if we are one of those for whom love does not come naturally, it can happen. God never created a soul that could not love him. It means putting aside negative thoughts like, "I can't love God."

It used to be that there were times when I would say to myself, "I love the Lord," and immediately a little voice inside me said, "No, you don't. You're not the type." It was a bit of old programming stuck in my brain, but I listened to it for quite some time. Finally one morning at five when I was working a jigsaw puzzle because I couldn't sleep, I realized what was happening. I said back to that little voice, "I am too the type. I love the Lord." I haven't heard that particular negative message since. I can say it. I love the Lord.

Mental illness changes the family dynamics. Consider the "possessed" boy [Mark 9:14-29]. The father told Jesus, "It has often thrown him into fire and into water to kill him." The father feared for the boy's very life. Possibly in his fear he kept the boy away from fire and water at all times, even when the boy was apparently well. Depending on how much insight the boy had into his illness, he may not have understood why the father restricted him, and may have assumed that the father did not want him to be warm or to be clean. The father, on his hand, fearing that the illness might kill his son, may have been over-protective.

This is all supposition which is not part of Scripture, but it illustrates how mental illness can affect the family dynamics and bring about tensions between well-meaning people, whether parent-child, spouse, or sibling. Relationships with our family members run the gamut from abandonment to support to suffocating. It becomes a problem when they are over-protective, not willing to let go so that we can make our own wellness choices. It may become necessary to wall off certain aspects of our lives. For example, my doctor doesn't know my maiden name, and my family doesn't know my doctor's name. There can be no breach of confidentiality.

Our life decisions—where to live, what to wear, what to eat, and even what mental health services to receive—are made by us as adults within our financial constraints. We may choose to involve others in those decisions, but we must retain ownership of those decisions. The exceptions are those times when we lose capacity to make reasonable decisions, for example when we are having serious suicidal thoughts. Then by court order others will step in and make decisions for our safety. This happens a very small per cent of the time. Having a mental illness does not by definition make us incapable of owning our decisions, and we have the legal right to make our own decisions.

A supportive family can be a wonderful asset, and those families who themselves are getting education and support seem best able to fill that role. Some go to family support groups in the hospital. When a person is out-patient, the family can connect with NAMI (National Alliance for Mentally Ill). It has chapters nationwide.

Does being mentally ill mean one came from a "bad" or dysfunctional family? No more so than having asthma or any illness. Genetics may be a factor. However, if a person with mental illness did happen to come from a family background that was deficient or not supportive, it means that person will have one more barrier to deal with on the road to recovery. It is not insurmountable. Many have done it. We can't blame others for who we are. We have the choice to change. As Thomas Merton said, "How do you expect to arrive at the end of your own journey if you take the road to another man's city?"[5] Or looking to St. Paul,

> ... you should put away the old self of your former way of life, corrupted through deceitful desires, and be renewed in the spirit of your minds, and put on the new self, created in God's way in righteousness and holiness of truth.

> Ephesians 4:22-24

Spouse, significant other.

In deep depression, other persons seem to be on the periphery of our struggle for existence. We don't see them clearly. Depression is hard on a marriage. I'm just not fun any more. My spouse feels resentment. How dare I withhold the part of me that's fun? He takes me out to dinner. That's supposed to fix everything. He's sincerely trying. I'm still depressed in the morning.

We might be pulling on the fabric of our relationships more than we need to. It is easy to become self-absorbed, to talk about how we are feeling and what we are experiencing to the exclusion of anything else. We listen less. We notice others' needs less, and—sadly—we even care less. We are the "sick" ones. We want people to help when there is nothing that can help. The illness becomes a third party to the relationship like an adulterous lover. There is a tendency to want to say, "I'm the one who is sick. I'm the one who should be getting chicken noodle soup." Some of that anger we feel at being sick gets displaced toward other persons in very subtle ways.

The fact is that, in such a relationship, when one is sick, all are hurting. It becomes necessary to learn to minister to each other alternately or even concurrently if the relationship is to survive. The following is from the unpublished novel *Clare Doe*. Clare has been discharged from her third psychiatric hospitalization in as many years, and her husband Frank is driving her home.

> He next spoke half a mile from home, passing the lilypad pond where she sometimes wound up on her walks. "I want a divorce."
>
> Clare let the words hang in the air so she wouldn't have to take them in, longed for the familiar faces of the hospital staff.
>
> "You are after all seriously ill. You showed that this past hospitalization. You always had something new to fight about whenever I stopped by."
>
> Pulling her feet up onto the edge of the car upholstery, Clare rested her arm across her knees, her

head on the arm as she looked out the side window away from him.

"This has been endless," he droned on. "And it looks like it will be endless. I want to live, not be tied to someone who is sick. Do you hear me? I want to live."

Clare still didn't answer. Frank pulled over to the side of the road, one side of the car resting in the weeds, the other in the gravel on the edge, the engine still running. The house was still out of sight, just beyond the next rise in the road. "How do you feel about this?" he asked.

Clare knew that he was bracing himself for the inevitable rebuttal, that he wanted to debate as they always did so he could prove his point, so that he could best her in a verbal skirmish and know for sure he had been right. She let a car go by before she answered. "I hurt all over," she said.

Frank drummed the steering wheel and opened his mouth as though to answer, but the only sound he made was a smacking noise with his lips. The motor's fan kicked on. Clare knew she didn't have to sit there, knew the house was just over the rise, but she waited.

Again he opened his mouth and closed it. Another car passed by, nobody that Clare recognized.

"That's all you have to say?" he asked.

"All." She pulled herself tighter into a ball on the seat.

"All right then." Frank put the car back into gear and pulled back onto the road without checking the mirror.

Clare Doe, unpublished

As the novel progressed, Frank relented later that evening, deciding to give her another chance since she had just got out of the hospital. Clare thought the whole episode very unfair. Hadn't he promised to love her in sickness and in health? It wasn't her fault she was sick.

The marriage eventually crumbled. Had Clare been able to hear Frank's very real pain instead of fixing on the injustice—an injustice to both of them—could the marriage have been saved? This excerpt is fiction, and in fiction one can have whatever ending one wants.

> Two are better than one: they get a good wage for their labor. If the one falls, the other will lift up his companion. Woe to the solitary man! For if he should fall, he has no one to lift him up. So also, if two sleep together, they keep each other warm. How can one alone keep warm? Where a lone man may be overcome, two together can resist. A three-ply cord is not easily broken.

Ecclesiastes 4:9-12

Children.

If the marriage stays together, then the family can stay together. If the marriage splits up, what becomes of the kids?

Some people with mental illness can function successfully as single parents, but the courts tend to have a bias against them. Some people quite honestly cannot cope and wind up losing their kids to Children's Services. There is only one hard and fast rule: If at all possible, the kids should have access to both parents without being placed in the middle, without fights because somebody was late, without games. Time with kids is healing.

My ex and I fought over money, and we fought over the desk, but by the grace of God we didn't fight over the kids. I didn't have custody, but the judge ordered frequent and liberal visitation. We set up a schedule so we would know what to expect, and we varied it when we needed to. The bottom line is that the kids always knew they had two parents who loved them, who supported the other parent's need to love them, and they turned out pretty well. I've never asked them about their experience of my illness, their fears and frustrations and even anger. I've always been afraid to.

Other relationships.

Friends/Siblings. Like Job's friends, our contemporaries mean well, but they may not understand our pain. Even if we try to tell them, they may not understand. They might encourage us to pick ourselves up by our bootstraps. They may tell us that we look okay to them, even though they are trying to understand.

One-sided relationships. "Therapeutic" relation-ships—psychiatrist, psychologist, counselor, case manager, spiritual guide—tend to be one-sided. Such people bring a certain knowledge and expertise which can give them an aura or mystique. Typically we make appointments and pay them for their services. It can be a powerful, even dependent relationship, and we must choose with care the person we put in this role. When it has been a good relationship, it has been beneficial toward my healing.

Community relationships. We can have a relationship with a civic organization or a day center or a workplace, to name a few. The people constituting it come and go over time, but we keep coming, because our relationship is with the organization, not with the individual people who make it up. A church can be a community relationship, or it can be a place to receive sacraments.

Forgiveness.

We can't discuss relationships without looking at forgiveness. We needn't worry about whether God forgives us. He is always willing to take us back. Whether others forgive us for our hurts to them is ultimately up to them. We can't control that. Our concern is with forgiving those who have hurt us, letting go of our anger. The bad news is that it is difficult to forgive. The good news is that it is easy. The bottom line is that it is essential to our own healing if not to the healing of a relationship. When I am angry, whether consciously or subconsciously, it seems to take a lot of my mental energy in the same way that a cold robs me of physical energy.

Anger is part of our emotional package as humans. St. Paul wrote, "Be angry, but do not sin; do not let the sun set on your anger, and do not leave room for the devil." [Ephesians 4:26-27]

Forgiveness is easy.

We have a lot of fixed notions about forgiveness, most of them impediments to reaching a state of forgiveness and healing. Consider a person who has done us wrong. It could be someone with whom we are in relationship (family, friend, colleague, neighbor). It could be the stranger who mugs us in the park. It could even be a loved one who has died. Anger is a stage of grief.

It is okay to be angry, and to say we are angry, but our thoughts often start going in the following unproductive circles:

I can't forgive him until he apologizes (false).

I can't forgive her until she has made it up to me (false).

I can't forgive him until he has been punished (goes to jail, loses his job, loses money, is cut off from seeing the kids) (false).

I can't forgive her until I "get the anger out" by telling my therapist, her best friend, and everybody at work (false). (Some of this helps, but there are times when it becomes spiteful and even addictive.)

⅄ What a lot of baggage we carry, our own individualized rules of fairness. We can't forgive unless it is "fair" by our rules.

⅄ Nobody apologized to Jesus when he was on the cross. They taunted and jeered at him, yet he said, "Father, forgive them; they do not know what they are doing." [Luke 23:34]

⅄ Forgiveness isn't fair or equalizing. Forgiveness is giving—freely giving. We are so steeped in our traditions of having things fair and getting even and saving face that we have lost sight of the goal to cleanse our own souls. We are called to forgive—either in person or from a safe distance—and move on. It is about following Jesus:

> And to another he said, "Follow me." But he replied, "[Lord,] let me go first and bury my father." But he answered him, "Let the dead bury their dead. But you, go and proclaim the kingdom of God."
>
> Luke 9:59-60

✳ This is a difficult passage. We are called to forget what is holding us back—many times our own lack of forgiveness—and move on. We are called to put aside all the structure we have built around forgiveness. To forgive is easy. We just do it. We don't wait for an apology. We just let go. The reward is great.

Forgiveness is difficult.

I am now going to contradict myself. Forgiveness is difficult. The choice to forgive is easy. It means mentally deciding to let go of the anger. Unfortunately the heart is slow to follow where the mind has chosen to go. We've decided to forgive, but then the anger creeps up again.

I know a psych nurse who said that hurt was just a polite term for anger. I played with the word "hurt," applying it to different contexts, but the bottom line was always that I was angry. In our anger we pray to God to take care of our sense of injustice:

> Break the arms of the wicked and depraved;
>> make them account for their crimes;
>> let none of them survive.

Psalm 10:15

✳ We have to remember to allow for God's will to be done. God moves in ways we cannot see, and one of his ways is to show mercy. For example, one day the Pharisees brought to Jesus a woman caught in adultery. Mosaic law said that the couple should be stoned to death. [Deuteronomy 22:22]

But when they continued asking him he straightened up and said to them, "Let the one among you who is without sin be the first to throw a stone at her." Again he bent down and wrote on the ground. And in response they went away one by one, beginning with the elders. So he was left alone with the woman before him. Then Jesus straightened up and said to her, "Woman, where are they? Has no one condemned you?" She replied, "No one, sir." Then Jesus said, "Neither do I condemn you. Go, [and] from now on do not sin any more."

John 8:7-11

People have hurt us. Have we never hurt anyone, intentionally or otherwise? Are we so good that we can throw the first stone? Forgiveness begins when we recognize our own imperfections. At the same time, we must forgive ourselves for those imperfections. God already has. Whether I consider myself hurt or angry, the goal is forgiveness.

Then Peter approaching asked him, "Lord, if my brother sins against me, how often must I forgive him? As many as seven times?" Jesus answered, "I say to you, not seven times but seventy-seven times."

Matthew 18:21-22

That's a lot of times to forgive someone. It's a symbolic number, not to be taken literally. For instance, once when I was dealing with a major hurt, I started saying the name of the person involved every day when I said the Our Father, when I got to the part, "as we forgive those who trespass against us." I was trying to make a deliberate choice to forgive. I think I did that for about two years, which would be 730 days. The hurt is finally gone. I feel okay about that person. I feel more healed.

We pray for the grace to forgive, even when it means praying 77 times or 7 x 70 = 490 times or more. When we pray for healing, God nudges us. "What about forgiveness? Are you going to pray to forgive, so your heart may heal?"

Solitude.

Solitude is a relationship in itself. It is more than the absence of companionship. Like darkness, the absence of light, solitude is in itself a tangible presence. I have a love-hate relationship with aloneness. During a busy day, I look forward to the time when I can come home, take in the welcome mat, and put on my pajamas.

Outside I can hear a dog barking, the maintenance guy mowing the grass. Inside all is still. Nothing happens unless I make it happen. There is no spontaneous action to cause my reaction, no hungry kids telling me it is time to cook, nobody asking me how my day was. I know Jesus is present, but he isn't sitting on the couch conversing with me. As I slide the cooking bag from freezer to microwave, I turn the radio to a talk show. They are discussing the Bengals' latest draft picks—franchise players all.

We get into a relationship with solitude. It can feel peaceful, or it can make me edgy. We have to work on our relationship with solitude as with any other relationship. Yet the Lord is present, not on the sofa but in a sense of reassurance. He will not abandon me. If one could describe in words the sense of the Lord's presence, there would perhaps be no atheists left. We have to believe what we cannot see, a sense of alone but not alone. I am reminded of the storm at sea, when Jesus was asleep in the boat [Luke 8:23-24].

> You are my help: do not cast me off;
> do not forsake me, God my savior!
> Even if my father and mother forsake me,
> the LORD will take me in.

Psalm 27:9b-10

Or in the words of an Islam mystic:

> Oh, my Lord, the stars are shining
> And the eyes of men are closed.
> Kings have shut their doors
> And every lover is alone with his beloved,
> And here I am alone with Thee.

As quoted in a publication of St. Leo Abbey

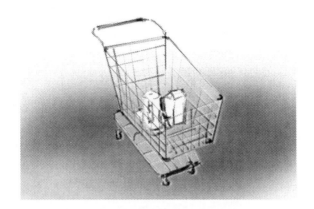

9. Coping.

To cope is to tread water. I splash about, stroking with my arms, kicking with my feet, with the goal of staying above water, of avoiding being overwhelmed. Getting to shore is another phase called recovery. For the time being I concentrate on treading water, on coping, on learning the survival skills. I offer here some of the coping mechanisms I have learned. Just as God's book deals with practical matters such as when to wash or what to eat, we deal here with practical advice on coping with depression.

The first step is to recognize what's broken. I have to realize that if I am fighting the same old battles in the same old ways, I will get the same results.

There was a time when I had trouble getting to the grocery. I would put it off until I was out of something crucial. Then I ran in for one or two items. The next day I found myself running in for something else. I was spending more time and energy going to the grocery than if I'd done a full shopping regularly, and I was getting frustrated besides.

I decided to do something about it. I decided that any

time I went to the store, I would get supplies for at least a week.

I decided to go at 3 p.m., but then it got to be 4 and the store is terribly crowded from then until after 6 but it's best not to go on an empty stomach so I should wait until after supper but 7 moved on to 8 and it's getting late so I should just run in for the bread and paper towels this time.

I had decided to change the way I shopped, but I hadn't actually changed anything. Same input, same outcome. I had to take a look at what was happening. The procrastination was because I didn't want to do it, and the reason I didn't want to do it was because there was some anxiety involved. I had to come up with some coping mechanisms to address the anxieties:

- If I needed a list to remember particular items, I made it in the morning or even the night before, but not as part of the process of getting out the door. The list helps with memory and decision-making functions and thus reduces anxiety.
- I have simplified my meal plan so that there are fewer decisions to make.
- I usually shop on Monday. Habit is powerful. The store is also less crowded.
- I leave the cart at the end of the aisle to avoid mid-aisle bottlenecks. I walk down for what I need and then move the cart to the next aisle.
- I thank God when it's done.

I didn't hit upon all of these modifications at once. They evolved over time, and they work. If the problem persisted, I could have looked for more imaginative solutions. In some cities the grocery stores deliver for a fee. It might be possible to hire a neighborhood teenager. For some people running in for a few things every other day is their best solution. Whatever works.

> When the just cry out, the LORD hears
> > and rescues them from all distress.
> The LORD is close to the broken-hearted;
> > saves those whose spirit is crushed.

> Psalm 34:18-19

Decision-making.

I once watched a bright young engineer spend two hours a day trying to fill out his hospital menu. My experience with decision-making while depressed is that one can't get all of the pieces of the decision into one's mind at the same time. It's like a computer with a very small RAM. I can load in the reasons for something, or the reasons against, but I can't put them in simultaneously to compare them side-by-side. I can't hold it all in my head. Here again, paper and pencil can help by listing reasons for and against.

Another tool is to downgrade the decision. Is the fate of the world resting on my choice? The impaired sense of time is making this seem of critical importance. At that particular moment, whether to choose peas or corn becomes an over-riding issue. I have lost perspective. I need to step back. Will this decision have ramifications in ten years? In ten days?

Another trick is to go for first acceptable rather than best possible. I see peas on the grocery shelf. Peas are okay. I buy peas. This requires a little bit of detachment, but it works also for clothes and other purchases. Does it meet my basic criteria? Then I don't need to confuse myself by looking further.

Some (but not all) choices have moral value. If I am trying to decide whether to serve peas or corn, say, to a spouse or to a guest, it doesn't much matter. But if I know my guest loves peas and hates corn, and I choose corn because I am in an ugly, spiteful mood, then I have made the wrong choice.

When Nicodemus visited Jesus at night, Jesus told him,

> "For everyone who does wicked things hates the light and does not come toward the light, so that his works might not be exposed. But whoever lives the truth comes to the light, so that his works may be clearly seen as done in God."

> John 3:20-21

The important decisions are those between light and dark, between good and evil. The decision is not always about what we choose to do, but how we choose to do it.

Memory.

My mind feels like an abandoned junkyard, rusting hulks of cars piled one upon another, scrap metal and broken glass, and I can't find anything useful. I certainly forgot things before the illness, but I'd misplaced them in my head. Now they go completely outside of my head, way beyond Pluto somewhere. Gone.

At work I use contact manager software to help me remember phone calls. At home I use mind manager software to help me remember what to write and what's been written. I have read books on improving memory with moderate success.

I use deliberate memory jogs. If I need to remember to take a book back to the library, I leave the book by the door where I will have to step over it to get by it. If I want to remember something refrigerated that I can't leave at the door overnight, I put my keys in the refrigerator. And of course I use lists. To-do lists both at work and at home, grocery lists, lists upon lists, and I still come home from the store without light bulbs. Then I have to try to use a sense of humor and be amused by myself rather than be frustrated. People do forget things.

It's okay to say, "I forgot," no excuses, no alibis, no lies to cover up. It's true that everybody forgets. I don't have to tell them it went past Pluto. Even when embarrassed, I own up to my deficiency so we can move on from there. Trying to fake my way through rarely works. I'd rather be seen as forgetful than dishonest.

Occasionally I surprise myself by remembering something I would have thought forgotten, like a name on a document from several months ago. It gives me hope that my head is steadily healing, and that the challenges of work are helping to improve it.

Before I bemoan my fickle memory, I have to affirm to how much is still working. Do I see my head as half empty or half full? With a few coping mechanisms, I can get by. Thanks be to God.

Fears and anxieties.

All of my fears are real events. Their basis may not appear real to others. If I am in a shopping mall and the walls are closing in, I feel fear. That is real to me. Perhaps nobody else at that time is experiencing a sense that the walls are closing in, but it is real to me. Something is happening to me. Call it misfiring brain cells. Call it shadows of nasty ideas emerging from the subconscious. Call it what you will, it is real in my world, and I am afraid.

I think of anxiety as being more faceless than fear. I am afraid of the sagging ceiling. When I am anxious, I don't know the cause. It is a dread I don't understand. Washing my hair makes me anxious, and I don't know why. For everyday hygiene I can take a quick bath in the evening, but whether I shower or sit in the tub and use the handheld attachment, I get anxious about washing my hair. I procrastinate for hours. I make myself more miserable until finally I do it. One would think that with repeated successes the anxiety would subside, but I go through the same drill each time.

I can think of instances—less frequent now—when I was attacked by feelings of anxiety for no apparent reason. Perhaps it was an adjustment to the changes that had taken place, changes in the ways I could or couldn't do things, even changes in the way I see things. I'm much less visibly perceptive. If I bounced along trying to be the old me, I would bump up against the changed parameters of the new me and experience internal conflict. Now I don't remember the old me. I am me.

In recent years I have been influenced by the model of the Wellness Recovery Action Plan (WRAP) developed by Mary Ellen Copeland. More information is available at www.mentalhealthrecovery.com. Some elements of my own plan:

- Prayer. "Please, God, help" is efficacious. I have favorite psalms (103, 91, 27, 121 to name a few) for such times. Other favorite passages of Scripture help.
- Doing something—walking, cleaning—can help. Conversely going to bed and concentrating on lying very still and redirecting my thoughts can help.
- Going to the zoo or the county park.
- Reading a novel or other diversions, like computer games.
- Calling somebody. If it has overwhelmed me and threatens to drown me, I can call the nearest professional, probably my doc. Other choices are suicide hotline or warmline. With other close people I can talk about my anxiety, but I have to be willing to move out of it to a general conversation.
- Meds. I take an antipsychotic medication, and I have permission to take a little extra as needed. I see it as a last resort used at most once or twice a year. Some other medications used for anxiety are addictive, that is, more and more does less and less.

Time is the key ingredient. Most spells of anxiety don't last forever. None of the above coping mechanisms brings instant relief. I may read for a while until the panicky feelings distract me too badly, and then switch to a phone call or a computer game or some tidying up, all interspersed with talking to God. If I keep stringing together enough coping activities, in time I will have out-lasted the bad feelings. And in time—over the years—they have become not a problem, only whispers when I am particularly stressed out.

> Why are you downcast, my soul;
>> why do you groan within me?
> Wait for God, whom I shall praise again,
>> my savior and my God.

Psalm 42:6

Articulation.

I remember during my fifth or sixth hospitalization sitting on a piano bench next to a young man whose hair was falling in his eyes after a two-month stay. He talked about the difficulty he had in making simple conversation. I nodded and said to him, "It's like the little place in my head that used to hear things before I said them is gone." He said to me, "Yeah, that's it. Finally somebody has described it."

Speaking is a little like flying by the seat of my pants. I open my mouth and out come words. Often I plan ahead what to say if I know I will be in a certain situation such as making a particular phone call, but that can lead to racing thoughts as it goes through my mind over and over. The best solution I have found is to try to feel good about people so that what comes out will be good.

> I said "I will watch my ways,
> lest I sin with my tongue;
> I will set a curb on my mouth."
> Dumb and silent before the wicked,

I refrained from any speech.
But my sorrow increased;
my heart smoldered within me.
In my thoughts a fire blazed forth,
and I broke into speech.

Psalm 39:2-4

Sleep.

As with many people with a bipolar illness, sleep or its lack can be a problem more at some times than at others. While some people have difficulty falling asleep, I have more trouble staying asleep. One rule of thumb I have is not to stress out about the fact that I'm not asleep. That only makes it harder to get back to bed. Some other things I have learned:

• A fixed bedtime and getting-up time establishes a pattern.

• I rest at intervals, but I avoid a pattern of day-sleeping. An occasional nap to take the edge off exhaustion can actually help sleep, but a pattern of daily naps only breaks down the amount of deep, uninterrupted sleep I get.

• Bedtime is not the time to mull over what's bothering me. If I need that time, then I have to shut off the radio, etc., at some point earlier in the evening to think things through. Committing the problem to paper in some fashion—even garbled notes—and leaving it there helps to take the problem out of my mind.

• Hospitals always taught us relaxation techniques. They had us lie on the floor on our backs and successively tense and relax each set of muscles, starting with the toes. Invariably some people fell asleep before the exercise was done. I feigned sleep so I could stop.

• If I am restless, I seek out pleasant thoughts as I try to fall asleep. In my head I visit my "green places" —memories of picnics or walks in the woods or other natural settings.

• Some listen to soothing music. I usually fall asleep around the seventh inning of the ball game (with apologies to Joe Nuxhall).

• Sometimes I just try to place myself in God's presence. Occasionally I use a mantra, concentrating on the words "Jesus, Lamb of God."

• I'll admit I abuse caffeine, and that doesn't help. It is a weakness of mine. I try to switch to decaf tea when it is late.

Some may not agree, but I think it best not to discuss sleep problems with anyone except a doctor, and even then only if I am asking for help. It gets to be self-martyrdom. ("Oh, I didn't sleep at *all* last night.") The attention received in itself becomes a reason for sleeping less. Instead I inhabit my funny 3 a.m. world alone, reading or doing the crossword puzzle from the newspaper, enjoying the stillness but knowing that I will pay in the morning. There's a fine line between can't sleep and won't sleep.

> I am like a desert owl;
>> like an owl among the ruins.
> I lie awake and moan;
>> like a lone sparrow on the roof.

Psalm 102:7-8

Getting up in the morning.

Let's face it. We have days (or weeks or months) when it is difficult to get out of bed. My head is heavy. It feels best on the pillow. That's a physical reality. The problem is that it doesn't get better while I am down. It is in making the effort to get going that my head finally starts to clear. It is a small act of faith.

I find it best to start gradually with a cup of coffee and a little Scripture. Movement helps to get the blood going. A little radio helps. Breakfast. Slow progress in getting going, like working out a charley horse. I set my alarms enough ahead to allow for my gradual emergence from subconsciousness. Getting up becomes such habit that I can do it in my sleep.

Currently I get up to go to work. At other times my reason for getting up was to get the kids to school or to go to the daily mass or a class I was taking or a day program. I believe that God has always had a door open somewhere, and there has always been a motivation to get going when I needed one.

Look and see.

When I played Scattergories with the kids, the game would require us to find something in the room beginning with the letter "D" (for example). It is amazing the things one notices when looking at the room with new eyes: door, doormat, daisy (in a picture), doily, dishes, dust.

I try to do this in my apartment. Look and see. What is out of place? What have I been stepping over or moving aside without noticing? What can I pick up and put away (or throw away) quickly and easily? Even if I only dispose of a few items per look, it is progress in that relentless task of keeping my living space livable.

I've heard some recommend taking everything that is out of place in a room and putting it in a laundry basket, and then putting it away from there. At least it gathers the items. My fear would be that there would always be half a basket of things that I didn't know what to do with. On the other hand, maybe those are the things I don't need.

Look and see. What is in need of cleaning? I can't expect to get it all done at once, but when I pick out the most critical (say the bathroom sink or the living room carpet) and get it done, I have made progress. People who haven't experienced it don't realize the type of concentration and mental energy needed for simple cleaning. However, illness is not a reason for not doing. It is a reason for adapting how we do things.

Weight management.

I gained significant weight gradually after the initial break. Some blame the meds. I don't know. My whole being slowed down. I indulged more in comfort foods. It all added up, so to speak.

When I finally became alarmed over my weight, I started praying each time I stepped on the scale, "Lord, please help me with my weight," and went on with my lifestyle. However, things changed around me. The diner where I ate my high-carb lunch closed, and I started packing a less-caloried lunch. Moves both at home and at work meant more stairs more often in the day. I began to see a little movement in the stubborn red line on the scale.

Did God close the diner so that I could lose weight? Actually the owner closed it because of problems in the neighborhood. But by my prayers I was predisposed to take advantage of the opportunity to change my eating habits. Similarly my workplace's move to a three-story building was for business reasons, but I opted not to use the elevator.

Encouraged by my early losses, I made more change. I call it the tweak method. My eating habits were fairly stable. I tended to eat the same kinds of foods for each meal. Rather than make a radical change all at once as happens when one "goes on a diet," I tweaked a few calories out of one meal, waited a while, then tweaked a few calories out of another. For example, for breakfast I substituted spinach salad with fat-free dressing for frozen waffles smothered in butter. A month or so later I substituted a gardenburger patty for the pasta accompanying the veggies in my evening meal. It was not a diet but a change in lifestyle, and I lost much of the weight. So far I have managed to keep most of it off, even though I have added back a few calories. I still pray when I get on the scale, because I know how easy it is for one's weight to creep up.

Movement/exercise.

I used to put exercise on my daily list of things to do. I very rarely checked it off, but I always put it there as a reminder that it was a goal, however abstract.

Exercise is good. It burns calories. It strengthens our hearts. It makes us feel better. It is a natural antidepressant. We can exercise at home, go to a gym and work out, or walk/jog/swim. If we can get ourselves to do it. That's a big "if." I have phases when I do regular floor exercises, and phases when I drop them. I even had a treadmill at one time.

To be depressed is to feel ennui, lassitude. We can't always get ourselves to do exercise. That realization was when I substituted the word "movement" on my to-do list. If I couldn't do what I needed most, I would substitute what worked.

Movement can be gentler. It is putting a tape in the player and dancing to the music, or merely swaying with it. It is walking or even strolling in a park, the neighborhood, or the mall. It is touching my toes when I am heating water in the microwave for instant coffee. It is making an extra trip to consult someone at work rather than picking up the phone.

Smoking cessation.

They say that the consumer rate of smoking is two or three times that of the general population. I have smoked for all of my adult life. For a while I couldn't even pray for God to help me stop. I was afraid he would answer, and I felt I couldn't live without cigarettes.

I have at least got to the point where I pray to be able to quit. I have cut back a little. I have not yet tried group, patch, hypnosis, or meds. Maybe I will. God heard my prayer on my weight, and I believe he will hear my prayer in this case, by whatever means.

Support.

Change thrives on involving other people. The classic example is Alcoholics Anonymous, a successful model where the meetings are an integral part of the program. The makers of smoking cessation products advertise that the success rate increases with involvement in a stop-smoking group. At home, I pick up when someone is coming over.

We run along in ruts, some better than others. When we decide to make a change, for example to exercise every afternoon, or to read Scripture every morning, or to give up dessert, we are going along on new terrain. The rut was much easier, and the temptation is to slip back into the rut. Eventually we will create a new habit, but in the meantime it is helpful to have one or more persons who are involved. It stops being my private endeavor and becomes a somewhat public event. It is easy to allow myself to fail privately, but more difficult to fail in public. I feel good about what I am doing when others are cheering me on.

Coping.

Coping is about a sequence of habit and change, habit and change. The habit makes a life activity manageable. Once the habit is established, once the things gets done or faced or managed on a regular basis, then change is possible, a small tweak in the direction of growth, of expanded horizons, of movement toward recovery. A new habit is established and assimilated, followed by another small increment of change in that or another area, another small leap into faith, another step toward recovery. It is not an overnight process, and it is not linear. Setbacks happen. Yet we have time, and God is leading us.

A voice cries out:
In the desert prepare the way of the LORD!

Make straight in the wasteland a highway for our God!
Every valley shall be filled in,
every mountain and hill shall be made low;
The rugged land shall be made a plain,
the rough country, a broad valley.
Then the glory of the LORD shall be revealed,
and all mankind shall see it together;
for the mouth of the LORD has spoken.

Isaiah 40:3-5

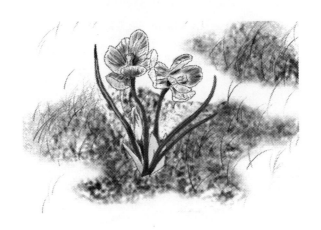

10. Healing.

I choose to use the word "healing" for its spiritual connotations. The word most common today is "recovery." Literally the word means to get back. If I lose my purse on the bus, I recover it when I get it back. Yet in healing we do not actually get back to where we were. Mental illness is a desert in our path of life, and we recover when we come out the other side and continue onward. I embrace the recovery concept. One also hears the word "resiliency," particularly with reference to children.

I had a significant recovery moment this past summer. I was driving home from a meeting of an advocacy committee in the state capital, and I was listening to an old tape I hadn't played in a while, *On Eagle's Wings* by Michael Joncas. When the title song came on, I remembered another time in another car in another state twenty years earlier.

It was August. I didn't know it, but I was already broken. By September I would be seeking a psychiatrist, but for the time being, I had bought time. I had dropped out of all the organizations I belonged to, and the pace of summer was easier.

My in-laws were having their annual family reunion, and it was up to me to drive the kids from our home on the East Coast to theirs in the Midwest. My husband was out of the country on business and would meet us there. I had a hard time concentrating on getting things pulled together and closing up the house, and we left three hours later than planned.

Once on the road, things went okay. The kids (ages 8, 6, and 4) were beautiful, chattering, napping, playing car games. I remember clearly a moment when rounding a long hill in Pennsylvania at about 5 p.m. Softly I sang to myself the refrain from "On Eagle's Wings," which I had learned only that summer. The verses are from Psalm 91, while the refrain reflects Deuteronomy. I felt supported, as though lifted up.

> As an eagle incites its nestlings forth
> by hovering over its brood,
> So he spread his wings to receive them
> and bore them up on his pinions.

Deuteronomy 32:11

How did I get from the hillside in Pennsylvania to a flat stretch on 1-71 twenty years later? A mile at a time. A step at a time. Jesus walked with me. I have no photographs to prove he was there. I can point to moments, like the day I saw a newspaper article about a clubhouse for people with mental illness that would help them get jobs. It turned out that there were three transitional employment slots for seventy people, but the structure and social interaction helped move me along.

A new door opened when I saw a notice posted for a ten-hour-per-week consumer position at yet another day program. Even though it wasn't enough to disrupt my benefits, I wasn't sure if I should take the plunge. I prayed at mass. A song that day was another favorite of mine, "Here I Am" by the St. Louis Jesuits which derives from Isaiah.

> Then I heard the voice of the Lord saying, "Whom shall I send? Who will go for us?" "Here I am;" I said; "send me!"
>
> Isaiah 6:8

I applied for the job and got it. I have to admit I haven't been employed continuously since. For a while I had to drop back to SSDI, but every experience eventually led to a new one.

Those twenty years were long years, and yet that moment in Pennsylvania seems as though it were yesterday. I didn't go back to the organizations I had dropped out of, as I had at first imagined I would. I am doing something new now. The kids are grown and gone. On the weekends they call me with their cell phones from the beach on the West Coast. The whole world has changed. And I am part of that world. That is recovery.

Jesus and healing.

Jesus came to proclaim the Kingdom of God, and by signs he indicated the nature of that Kingdom to come. He walked on the water once. He fed the multitudes twice. He healed hundreds, if not thousands, of times. After the beheading of John the Baptist,

When Jesus heard of it, he withdrew in a boat to a deserted place by himself. The crowds heard of this and followed him on foot from their towns. When he disembarked and saw the vast crowd, his heart was moved with pity for them, and he cured their sick.

Matthew 14:13-14

Jesus healed so that people may believe in this new kind of Kingdom. He quoted Isaiah in saying:

"The Spirit of the Lord is upon me;
> because he has anointed me
> to bring glad tidings to the poor.
He has sent me to proclaim liberty to captives
> and recovery of sight to the blind,
> to let the oppressed go free,
and to proclaim a year acceptable to the Lord."

Luke 4:18-19; cf. Isaiah 61:1

It is a Kingdom which is present but not yet actualized. For many people healing denotes making whole again, being restored to one's former state. A more realistic definition would be to say that healing means becoming functional again, useful in some capacity not necessarily related to our former purposes in life. It may or may not mean employment for wages, at least at first. It may mean a friendship, a usefulness to some other person.

Now that he is no longer physically with us, does Jesus heal in the present age, the Kingdom not yet realized? The glib assurances flow so easily from the pen. Of course he does, one wants to say. To give credibility to that answer is more difficult. I've heard of miracles, of complete and

117

sudden remission of symptoms for no discernible medical cause. I've never personally met someone who experienced such a miracle. I like to believe at least some of those instances are true, that God was moved to set aside his natural order for that one time. For most of us healing is more gradual, and it doesn't necessarily mean remission of symptoms.

I have a friend who years ago lost all his fingers except one thumb in an industrial accident. He can use the thumb, and he can grip between the tops of the knuckles so that he can do functions like writing and eating well. He says the only thing that is a problem is the very top button at his collar. He leaves that undone and pulls his tie up tight.

Long ago I was in the same organization as a woman who was blind from birth. With the help of adaptive mechanisms, she was able to support herself, and she was president of the organization's chapter in her town. When several of us from the organization went to a state meeting, we stayed at a motel which had rooms spread out over many levels in many corridors. We could follow the signs to the dining room, but we got confused about which way to go to get back to our rooms. My friend knew. She had trained herself to count all the twists and turns and to be able to reverse them in her head. It was a case of the blind leading the sighted.

Healing does not mean cure in the traditional sense. I can think of two excellent books, *The Gift of Peace* by Joseph Cardinal Bernardin and *Lessons from the School of Suffering* by Rev. Jim Willig, both written by priests who had cancer, both of whom succumbed to that illness. Nevertheless to read their books is to read of the healing they experienced in the journey to new life. It is all about the Kingdom.

Healing from mental illness is two-fold: alleviating negative symptoms and reembracing a positive life. Of the two, the former is easiest. We can learn to deal with symptoms by coping mechanisms, by medicating them away when necessary, or simply by accepting them and adapting. Many symptoms, such as anxiety or anhedonia ("glumness") merely go away over time. It has been said that the difficulty in recovery from mental illness lies not in the illness but in the social and psychological manifestations of the illness.

That brings us to the second phase, rebuilding a life. It can mean re-establishing old relationships that were strained during the tough times, or it can mean starting new relationships, or both. It can mean having a place to go on a consistent basis. It can mean having a function, a role. It can mean doing something for God.

For me, the key ingredients in my healing were (and still are) God, social interaction, and structure. I've found them in many places, including now at the workplace. The fact that I get paid for working, that I support myself, is an extra bonus. Often while he preached, St. Paul worked as a tentmaker:

> For we did not act in a disorderly way among you, nor did we eat food received free from anyone. On the contrary, in toil and drudgery, night and day we worked, so as not to burden any of you.
>
> 2 Thessalonians 3:7-8

The four-corner hole.

We all need healing in the various areas of our life—body, mind, heart, and soul—but we needn't do everything at once. Any healing of one area works for the benefit of all. If we feel a little better physically, we feel better in the other domains as well. If we lift our spirits, it improves our overall well being.

It is like a piece of fabric with a four-corner hole or a sock with a hole in the heel that needs to be darned. We can't begin to mend in the middle, for there is nothing to anchor to. If we put a few threads across the top, it makes the sides shorter and easier to work with. There is a lot of whole fabric left in the sock, but it is the hole which is most noticeable to us. If we put a patch on it, it will only tear more. We must reconstruct the cloth a thread or two at a time, one side at a time. Once we get going, it is a satisfying process, because we are working toward wholeness. Jesus said,

> "No one sews a piece of unshrunken cloth on an old cloak. If he does, its fullness pulls away, the new from the old, and the tear gets worse."

Mark 2:21

We don't take a patch of healing and sew it on our old lives. We use it to create new lives, to become new persons.

Healing takes effort. It takes exercise of body, mind, heart, soul, but effort in one domain will help the others. Also, an activity can be effort and fun at the same time. Some directions for exercising the whole of me:

My body says move. Do simple floor exercises. Use the stairs. Consider yoga or aerobics classes. Walk.

My mind says learn. Grow. Work puzzles. Do new things, or old things in a new way. One book I've enjoyed is *Keep Your Brain Alive* by Lawrence C. Katz, Ph.D., and Manning Rubin. It suggests such simple neurobic exercises as using the nondominant hand or taking a different route to work.

My heart says try to love. Try to forgive, and ask to be forgiven. Try to give to those in need, even a token amount. Stretch those heartstrings.

My soul says spend time with God. Pray. Read Scripture. Find an uplifting church.

Obviously these can be combined in any number of ways. For a while I went through a phase when I said a rosary as I walked (body and soul). I have made lists of what I've seen (or heard) on an outing (mind and body). I've said a silent prayer as I was talking with someone (heart and soul).

Waiting.

When I was a kid, I felt like I was waiting for my life to begin. I was in a preparatory phase learning the names of planets and the names of Presidents and taking music lessons. I spent easily the first two decades of my life waiting for life to begin. After I started family and work, I didn't think about it. I was deeply into life.

Then it stopped. Mental illness. For a time I again felt that I was waiting for life to begin, hoping that it would happen. Now I have become involved in life all over again. The wait was worth it.

The sense of healing is like the first full day of spring in mid-March. We are still packed into our winter coats for protection from the chill air. The sky is gray, and patches of snow linger under the trees. Yet on sunnier slopes, purple and yellow crocuses bloom, and we know that the worst is over. Better days are coming.

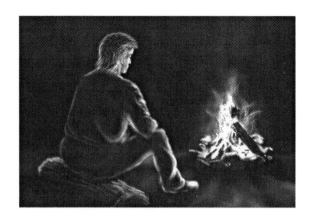

11. Where I found God.

The following realities have become clearer to me in my search for the God of the low places.

Depression is not my fault. It is not God's retribution for sin. It is an illness. Depression happens.

Recovery happens. God wants it to happen. God cares. God will hear me.

Jesus wants to heal me. I can help myself heal. Spend some time with Jesus. Spend some time with others.

Keep the faith.

Have hope.

Try to love.

Not only that, but we even boast of our affliction, knowing that affliction produces endurance, and endurance, proven character, and proven character, hope, and hope does not disappoint, because the love of God has been poured out into our hearts through the holy Spirit that has been given to us.

Romans 5:3-5

(Footnotes)

[1] Larson et al., "The Role of Clergy in Mental Health Care," in James K. Boehnlein, MD, ed., *Psychiatry and Religion,* American Psychiatric Press, Inc., 2000.

[2] St. Teresa of Avila, *The Life of Teresa of Jesus,* E. Allison Peers, trans., Image Books, 1960.

[3] *The Way of Perfection,* St. Teresa of Avila, E. Allison Peers, trans., p. 168.

[4] Martin Buber, "The Way of Man According to the Teachings of Hasidism," in *Religion from Tolstoy to Camus,* Walter Kaufman, ed., Harper & Row, 1961, p. 429.

[5] Thomas Merton, *Seeds of Contemplation,* page 61.

About the Author

The author has experienced first-hand the debilitating effects of depression. By the grace of God, she has now recovered sufficiently to work with and share the experiences of others with similar afflictions. She is a practicing Catholic, but the book is intended for a broad faith outlook.